Product of Misinformation

Demystifying Cosmetics and Personal Care Claims, Terms, and Ingredients

by
Michael Rutledge

Learn how to see through the absurd and
unbelievable claims of much of the industry,
and find a product that works for you

Also included, from the scientists who
research and formulate the products:
"The ten steps to sensible skin care."

Tapestry Press
Irving, Texas

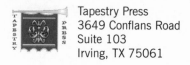

Tapestry Press
3649 Conflans Road
Suite 103
Irving, TX 75061

Printed in the United States of America

05 04 03 02 01 5 4 3 2 1

Library of Congress Cataloging-in-Publication Data

Rutledge, Michael Joseph, 1946-
    Product of misinformation : demystifying cosmetics and personal care claims, terms, and ingredients / by Michael Joseph Rutledge.
        p. cm.
Includes bibliographical references.
    ISBN 1-930819-14-5 (trade pbk. : acid-free paper)
    1. Cosmetics. 2. Hygiene products. 3. Consumer education. I. Title.
    RA778 .R965 2002
    646.7'2—dc21

                            2001008061

Notice

Nothing herein is warranted or guaranteed. Much constitutes the opinion of the author and fellow cosmetic chemists, based on their experience. For example, many of the uses of herbal extracts are anecdotal in nature. The safety of each formulation must be determined by the reader. Many of the examples given are several years old.

Book design and layout by
D. & F. Scott Publishing, North Richland Hills, Texas

Contents

Acknowledgments

The author wishes to thank everyone who contributed to this book, and in particular: chemists Neal Hutchinson and Kimberly Leahy for their expertise, help and opinions; Amy Davies for her research; Purity Life Health Products of Canada for the use of some of their definitions in the "Dictionary of Terms Used" section (they did a wonderful job of making them consumer-friendly); Elizabeth Fuller, who not only did the word processing but was forced to contend with my handwriting; and last, but not least, those who helped cover my duties at Earth Science, Inc. while I spent time on this manuscript.

Thank you all for your help.

Michael Rutledge
Earth Science, Inc.
475 N. Sheridan Street
Corona, CA 92880-9836

Preface

As I finish this book I am 54 years old, having spent all of my life since I was 17 in the laboratories and manufacturing facilities of various chemical, pharmaceutical and cosmetic companies. I can say without fear of regret that no industry in which I have been employed comes close to matching the misunderstanding of products and ingredients found in the personal care industry. Inferior products are sold via intentional misinformation, good products are hyped beyond belief and truly great products are promoted for reasons other than those that makes them great.

Is it the amount of competition? The desire to appear different? To cater to that very human urge to look better overnight (without too much effort, of course)? A pure appeal to vanity? The fact that regulation is lax in the area of "beauty" claims?

The answer is probably a bit of all of the above. Like obtaining good medical treatment, educating yourself is the only way to really understand what you are getting for your money. A byproduct of your education will be the understanding that not everything we put on our skin or hair is good for us. In fact, there are products in the marketplace that can endanger your long-term health.

This book is an attempt to get you started. For the serious among you who want to pursue your education, you can use the bibliography. There is not enough space in this volume to go into the physiology of the skin and hair, nor the complex nature of personal care formulating. If you want to understand formulating, my favorite book for that is:

Harry's Cosmeticology: Chemical Publishing
edited by Martin Rieger (New York: February 2000)
ISBN: 0-8206-0372-4

No doubt there will be chemists who say I have oversimplified the chemistry of it all. Likewise, some consumers may feel it is a bit too technical in places. I have tried to find the middle ground, based on my belief that given the facts in an understandable form, most everyone can make prudent decisions.

Preface

While it started out as an "ingredient dictionary," this text ended up as an attempt to motivate each reader to begin to "qualify" the companies from whom they purchase. Regardless of what the ingredient dictionary in chapter 7 says about a particular ingredient, clever, experienced, intelligent formulating can often overcome some of the negatives. Two different chemists can produce formulas with very different irritation potentials using many of the same ingredients, based on their skill and knowledge. It is up to you to get educated and find companies in whom you can build confidence. I can assure you that the amount of advertising money spent by a company is no indication of safety or concern for the consumer.

The purpose of this book is to help you see through the "clutter" and understand how to get to the facts. I hope you enjoy it.

Anatomy of the Skin

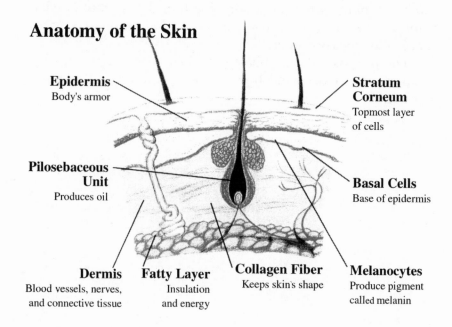

Epidermis
Body's armor

**Stratum
Corneum**
Topmost layer
of cells

**Pilosebaceous
Unit**
Produces oil

Basal Cells
Base of epidermis

Dermis
Blood vessels, nerves,
and connective tissue

Fatty Layer
Insulation
and energy

Collagen Fiber
Keeps skin's shape

Melanocytes
Produce pigment
called melanin

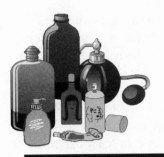

Chapter 1

Swimming in a Sea of Misinformation

"Unprovided with original learning, uninformed in the habits of thinking, unskilled in the arts of composition, I resolved to write a book." Edward Gibbon (1737–1794)

I did not want to write a book. The thought was frightening in its own way—long hours at the computer, less time in an already hectic life and sharp declines in the already strictly allocated hours available for research and product development.

I resisted the calls by our distributors and salespeople to set the public record straight. I attempted to ignore the ever-increasing customer requests for the first truly correct cosmetic ingredient dictionary. But the end of my resistance arrived with the growing flood of misinformation, incomplete explanations by certain authors and uneducated feature writers, and shameless distortions of truth by some companies. In short, it irritates me to read some of the so-called "ingredient explanations" and "ingredient dictionaries." At best, most of them are incomplete. Sadly, the majority are filled with inaccuracies and gross distortions of the facts.

Early on, I want to state for the record that proper skin and hair care can prevent premature aging, help keep skin and hair healthy and very effectively treat many common skin problems. I am convinced that it works well to alleviate and prevent many common skin ailments. Acne, "breakouts," psoriasis, dry skin, wrinkles, dandruff and so forth are all treatable, and in many cases preventable. I am a strong believer. There is ample scientific evidence in this respect. It is this fact that so frustrates chemists when inferior products (and sometimes exceptional products) are sold via misinformation.

There was a time when chemists used to laugh over the foolishness and sometime idiocy of the inaccuracies. Only when it became obvious to me that it would continue and gradually become the beliefs of many of our customers did I consent to write this text.

This book may not be what you've heard or read, but it's based on the latest scientific information available. If nothing else is remembered by the reader, the appendix will at least list some of the very best sources of information for future reference.

Why the Deluge of Misinformation?

Of course I can't know what is in the heart and mind of every marketing person or writer. I assume much of it is done in an honest attempt to educate the public. However, in tracing back many of the rumors and falsehoods, we have found the following items to be the all too frequent sources:

I   Labels, Company Brochures and Product Inserts

This is definitely not the best source of scientific knowledge available. Are you thinking "how could regulatory agencies permit less than the full truth on a package or in a brochure"?

The answer is that cosmetics[1] (non-pharmaceutical skin care, hair care, body and bath products, and color formulas) are provided different rules than their drug and food counterparts. The U.S. Food and Drug Administration (USFDA), whose responsibility it is to regulate these cosmetics, has less authority (and less interest) in body care. While much of this information refers to the USFDA, it also applies in most cases to Canadian law and that of other countries as well.

For example, in the case of cosmetics, they are essentially reduced to reviewing sanitation and good manufacturing procedures in the production facility. A secondary function is to review the label for *claims*. This "claim review" function concerns itself mainly with making sure that the cosmetic does not make "drug" claims. If it does, the product can be classified as a drug and

---

1   In this text we will use the term "cosmetics" to refer to all non-pharmaceutical skin care, body care, hair care, bath products, and color products.

recalled if it is not properly labeled as a drug (it is highly unlikely it would be properly labeled as a drug if the manufacturer believed it was a cosmetic). A "dandruff control" shampoo can be a cosmetic, while the same shampoo labeled as "anti-dandruff" can be classified as a drug. (I don't make the rules.)

This label review of a cosmetic rarely includes investigating the validity of the cosmetic claims. The attitude seems to be "If it's not making drug claims, it can say whatever the company desires." I'm sure you can see the opening here for unscrupulous marketers. In fact, the USFDA goes so far as to use the term "puffery" to describe this unregulated bloating of the facts. FDA Inspectors have told me that "puffery is expected" in the cosmetic business.[2]

A second reason for the lack of interest is a very enviable safety record by the cosmetic industry. When you consider the millions of products sold each year, the rate of safety issues is extremely low. The USFDA rightfully puts its limited resources to use where safety concerns are the highest—food, drugs and medical devices.

While the safety history is good, the industry's record on substantiating its claims is not something of which to be proud.

The label is good for "directions." Don't rely on it for real science. The brochure's purpose is to sell product. It is *not* your best source of facts.

II Magazine and Newspaper Articles

Sorry, these are little help to you beyond recommending a product for you to try. Hopefully, the author has previewed it for you and can give you his/her educated opinion.

Much (not necessarily all) of the information in these articles comes from a phone call to the manufacturer or distributor of the product. It may not be a shock to you, but manufacturers can "expand" the truth to favor their particular product. In fact, I have seen portions of some articles taken directly from the manufacturer's brochures we discussed in the paragraphs above.

---

2 Yes, especially if one has not taken the time to understand the science of formulating truly effective products. The FTC (Federal Trade Commission) does occasionally address false advertising claims, usually after a complaint from a competitor.

Another source of misinformation from these articles is the anecdotal comments included in them, with little or no scientific evidence. Examples of these are listed later, in chapter 2.

Sadly, much of what you read about personal care in magazines and newspapers is not only incorrect, but designed to promote products and ingredients for its advertisers, all without proper research by the writer. It is no coincidence that you often see an article raving about the wonderful qualities of ingredient "x," only to find an ad for a product with ingredient "x" in it on the very next page. I can assure you that this collusion does not result in all the facts being carefully reviewed and fully revealed.

III   The Attempt to Correlate Raw Material Data with Finished Product Data

I could write a book on this subject alone—the source of great frustration for customer service groups at most companies.

Sometimes it is intentional misinformation from an unscrupulous manufacturer who wants to make his own product look good, or more often, who is motivated to make someone else's look bad.

Other times it is clearly a misunderstanding on the customer's part of the *importance of concentration* of an ingredient in a formula.

The scenario usually goes like this:

(1) A customer calls, quite upset because he/she just "learned" that a certain ingredient ("x") can burn the eyes (or irritate the skin, or cause a rash, etc.)

He or she is usually outraged that manufacturers are allowed, or dare to use, such an item in a personal care formula.

(2) Upon investigation we determine that the customer has been given the data that is supplied *to* a cosmetic manufacturer, *from* the single ingredient (raw material) supplier. This material safety data sheet[3] (MSDS) is written for the purpose of telling the chemist how to handle the *pure* raw material during manufacture of a product. As an example, alpha hydroxy acids in their pure form can burn unprotected skin. The manufacturer needs to know this. Yet, *if*

---

3   Required for each ingredient sold to a manufacturer in the U.S.

formulated properly, they can be quite beneficial and completely harmless in the lower percentage found in some finished products.

As a second example, handling pure Vitamin C powder requires precautions not needed in finished Vitamin C products.

(3) This "pure raw material data" has been reported to the public as though every finished product containing it should be avoided. There is no correlation in the vast majority of cases. *You cannot use raw material data alone to evaluate finished products.* The safety (or lack thereof) must be determined on the finished mixture. Can you imagine the MSDS for pepper, and chilies? "Caution: Can burn the skin and eyes, can cause rashes, gastric distress, etc." Yet, properly "formulated," they can be quite beneficial and harmless (and tasty).

I would add, there are a few ingredients that should generally be avoided in almost any concentration above a trace amount. We will discuss those in the dictionary in chapter 7.

IV Books Like This One

Our company operates an "800" number (see appendix A) as a free service to the industry. While we will not field questions on specific products or brands, our laboratory will attempt to answer all ingredient questions—whether or not it is an ingredient in our formulas. If we cannot answer it on the phone, we will later fax or e-mail our findings to the customer. From this perspective, we have a picture window to view what is causing confusion for customers.

Without a doubt, the source of the vast majority of confusion about ingredients stems from the so called "ingredient dictionaries" already in print. Most are misleading, misinforming, incorrect, slanted and/or only partially true. They often give only a "hint" of a possible problem with no further explanation. An example of this kind of silliness is a phrase often used—"Can be toxic."

Can be toxic? What exactly does that mean? Should we stop using any product with that ingredient today? Toxic at any concentration? (Of course not.) Toxic in my favorite product? Do they mean just the pure raw material? Does my product contain the "toxic level?"

Do you see the flaw? It's just enough information to worry you, but not enough to make you knowledgeable. Kind of like the ads during a political election. It sells books, but does not help consumers. As consumers and readers, we have an obligation to recognize that wild statements about the dangers of ingredients may induce us to purchase a book purporting to warn us of the impending menace to our health. The real facts behind the issue may be somewhat less exciting.

I have yet to locate an accurate (or even mostly accurate) consumer ingredient dictionary, but please file this fact away for future use: *Every material on this planet "can be toxic" at some level.* Even water. The phrase, by itself, is meaningless.

V Price

Every *chemist* I've ever met wants to formulate the very best product she/he[4] can.

Alas, every *company* does not want the "best" product—they want the best product at the price they can afford to pay.

Now here is where it gets strange. You must repeat this absolute truth until you have it memorized:

> *"There is no direct relationship*
> *between quality and retail price"*

Corollary #1—Quality must be defined. We define it as a product that accomplishes two things:

♦ It does very well what it says it does and

♦ It is safe to use and not likely to cause a skin or scalp reaction. (Some allergic reactions will be unavoidable, even in safe, natural products.)

Corollary #2—Sometimes you do get what you pay for. There is a price below which no chemist can create a high quality product. It is safe to assume that $1.99 for 16 ounces won't buy you a truly great shampoo.

Corollary #3—If you use it and like it, it's a quality product.

Corollary #4—You cannot tell *quality or safety* simply by reading the ingredient list or looking at the retail price.

---

4 Many of the best chemists I have known are women. I did not want to put "he" first every time, lest I hear about it later.

Corollary #5—There is a way to determine a quality product (see chapters 3, 4 and 5).

You may have believed that a $30.00 product has a higher raw material cost than a $15.00 product. Maybe. Maybe not. Maybe the extra cost is because of all the $15,000 ads run in a series of magazines. (Yes, it does cost that much, and more, to run a single ad in some magazines.) You see, every company decides where to spend its money. Some choose ingredients, research and development. Some choose advertising. For most companies, it is a varying blend of both. Even great products need to be made known to the customer in some fashion. Repeat again;

> *"There is no direct relationship*
> *between quality and retail price"*

Much misinformation results from trying to compare prices and ingredient lists of products. More comes as a result of trying to determine the "ingredient safety" by reading or comparing those lists. It is not uncommon to see a label emblazoned with a phrase such as, "Contains the amazing ingredient (herb, vitamin, latest fad, etc.)," to get your attention. I can tell you from analyzing many of those products, that only microscopic quantities, if any, are normally present. This is usually done to get the consumer's attention and keep the cost low. That does not mean the price to the consumer will necessarily be low. In fact, claiming the product contains the latest "fad" ingredient is usually a reason to keep the price high, whether or not the ingredient had any substantial effect on the product cost.

Do not evaluate your products by the retail price or the ingredient list. You must be *very* knowledgeable to use ingredient lists to determine safety and quality.

VI   The Sound-Alike Syndrome

Non-technical people are often confused or misled by names that sound similar. In most cases they have no relationship to each other. If they do have a relationship, it is often misunderstood.

For example, "sodium lauryl sulfate" sounds close to "sodium laureth sulfate" and often the two are confused or believed to be the same.

The names are similar because they are close in molecular structure (chemists name ingredients based on molecular content, shape, size, and/or source). These ingredients, while both are cleansers, are quite different in cleansing power, foam, irritation potential, and other characteristics (and certainly different on a molecular level).

While chemists use this naming system, most of the time little can be concluded by a layperson from simply looking at the name. Small differences in molecules can mean huge differences in their properties.

In our example above:

"Sodium" means that it is a sodium salt ("Salt" does not mean table salt in this context—somewhat confusing in itself).

"Lauryl" means that the main molecular chain contains 12 carbon atoms and it is from lauryl (fatty) alcohol (not like grain alcohol—more confusion).

"Sulfate" means that the SO_4 group (composed of sulfur and oxygen atoms) appears on the end of this molecule—that's all it means—nothing else. There is nothing sinister about sulfate as a group. Some sulfates are good— some are not so good for your skin.

"Laureth" means that the "Lauryl" part of the molecule has been changed (to increase mildness and improve solubility in this case). It is now a new molecule.

Avoid trying to draw too many conclusions from similar-sounding names. It will fool you much of the time.

VII   Rumors

I have no idea who starts them or why. I'll address a couple of the strangest in chapter 2.

VIII   Confusion over Internal Use and External Use

It is abundantly clear that some cosmetic manufacturers are advertising the internal benefits of a particular ingredient, as though the product was designed to be ingested. They misunderstand (or intend to misinform) that some ingredients have different functions when taken internally versus application to the skin and hair. We also see this regularly in magazine articles intended for consumers (usually filled with inaccuracies).

The following is a list of just a few examples of ingredients with different purposes:

Ingredient	Internal Use	Cosmetic Use
Panthenol	"B" vitamin source	Skin moisturizer/ healing agent/hair conditioner/increases the volume of each hair
Retinyl Palmitate or Retinol	Vitamin A source and all related functions	Antioxidant, moisturizer, skin peeling agent, acne treatment
Amino Acids	"Building Blocks" of proteins—a variety of internal uses	Moisturizers, hair and skin conditioners
Niacin	"B" vitamin source	Capillary stimulator to increase blood flow in a localized area
Collagen	Source of protein and amino acids	Moisturizer; temporary skin firmer
Co-Enzyme Q-10	Heart health	Antioxidant

It's important to know the internal purpose of ingredients in our diet. It may, however, have nothing to do with their use in personal care formulas. On the other hand, ingredients such as antioxidants can have a similar effect internally and externally. Therein lies yet another reason for obtaining an informed, reputable source.

IX   Advertising and Our Own Desire for a "Quick Fix"

An advertising executive once told me that I should develop a product that "removes cavities from teeth." At first I laughed, before I realized her point. Nothing catches our interest more in an ad than a quick fix to an annoying problem. Sometimes we let logic be obscured by our desire to solve a problem without paying the required price or putting in the necessary effort. Removing a hole in a tooth by brushing is not beyond the realm of possibility in the advertising world.

If you think of it in these terms, its not so hard to understand why we seriously consider the $29.95 "magic miracle overnight wrinkle remover" we see on late night television.

Removing deep wrinkles from years of neglect is—like brushing away your cavities—not so easily solved. The good news is that both are preventable.

A magazine survey found that 40 percent of women who read cosmetic ads don't believe them. And I do not blame them. The true and valid claims are becoming obscured by the ridiculous, making it almost impossible for the consumer to sort them.

Use logic when listening to advertising. Don't believe everything you read. Yes, there are those who might deceive you or distort the facts.

One last thought about the misinformation concerning safety and ingredients. Whenever I speak on this subject, I can see the looks of confusion when I point out that the safety and effectiveness of a formula is the result of the *mix* of all the ingredients in a product. Once mixed, the safety of each ingredient alone is rarely any longer the sole determining factor. For example, sodium lauryl sulfate is a cleanser that when used alone, in high concentration, tends to "overclean" and "dry" the skin or scalp. However, it is possible to formulate a safe baby shampoo that contains sodium lauryl sulfate. It might be possible or even less expensive to do it that way, but it is much easier to use mild amphoterics like cocoamphocarboxyglycinate or some of the mild sulfosuccinate surfactants.

It is also possible to formulate a shampoo with sodium lauryl sulfate that badly irritates the eyes. Like most things in life, you need sources who know what they are doing. Good chemists, like good lawyers, doctors, and friends, remain a minority of their total population.

From whom are you getting your information? Manufacturers? Magazine articles? Rumors? Laypersons without adequate background? Find a source you can count upon to give you all the facts. Locate a company or two in whom you have confidence.

Now let's have some fun with those who misinform us.

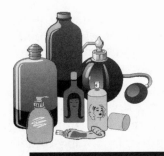

Chapter 2

Myths, Magic and Other Mendacities[1]

"Honesty is the best image." Ziggy (Tom Wilson)

I cannot possibly review every one of the thousands of examples of misinformation I have seen over the years. In this chapter we will take on a few (with the help and memory of several chemists who contributed to this book).

I Company Brochures and Labels

I like our own advertising agency people. They are fun to be around, outgoing, humorous and they always see things in a "media sort of way."

Marketing people are interesting, creative persons—artistic in their own way. They are not scientists, and the ones I know do not care to be such. They think of scientists as people too rigid to be creative—too concerned with facts to communicate well.

Their job is to determine the main selling points of a product and transform them into an interesting, easily understandable format for communication to the public. Sometimes it is their lack of understanding that causes them to not get the message completely correct. Sometimes the message is not unique enough and will be "expanded upon" by the marketing group in a desire to motivate the public. (I'm getting more tactful as I grow older.)

Let's get to it. Here are a few examples from company- produced brochures:

> *"Liposomes carry the active ingredients into the lowest layers of the skin."*

---

1   I've been waiting several months to find a use for that word.

11

This is not necessarily a good thing, but fortunately, most likely not true. The "lowest layers" would probably take the product into the bloodstream, certainly not the intention of any cosmetic. This is either a misunderstanding about skin physiology or an attempt to make the claim larger than reality. Liposomes can be very beneficial, but this claim is stretching the facts. Also, the "actives" to which the author is referring are a very important factor in measuring the actual skin absorption. (See "Liposomes" in the "Terms" section in chapter 6 of this book.)

This brings to mind a good question—are these claims of "deep penetration" just "puffery," or do these chemicals reach our bloodstream? No cosmetic product should be formulated for "absorption into the lowest layers of the skin." That would either be stepping into the drug arena or the result of poor formulation. A second reason to avoid deep penetration is that this dramatically increases the likelihood of irritation.

Experienced chemists are aware that certain ingredients (Vitamin A, for example) do tend to penetrate the skin well. Likewise, certain ingredients (propylene glycol, for example) tend to increase the penetration of other ingredients. There is no substitute for knowledgeable formulation, but regrettably, there are many formulas in the marketplace put together without this knowledge.

"Your skin's oxygen content may increase up to 100% in 12 to 14 days."

Not likely, but even if it miraculously accomplished that feat, the brochure gives no indication of how that could benefit you. The key word is "may." You will find "may," "helps" and "promotes" to be common hedge words in brochures. But it sounds good and it is nice marketing—a word with a positive connotation like "oxygen" must be good for you! One other thought—if antioxidants are good for you, and oxygen causes oxidation, isn't there a conflict in information?

"Less than 1% of antioxidants taken orally reach your skin."

When you see things like this, ask for a copy of the study (watch them squirm). There was no explanation of what percent might be okay or what antioxidants (since they differ so greatly) were in question, and definitely no explanation of how the 1 percent figure was obtained.

❀ ❀ ❀

"All natural—no preservatives."

This is a common claim but almost always untrue. Any formula with a significant level of water in it—whether the water be in pure form or as part of an infusion or extract —must be preserved. If not preserved, the product will spoil just as your food will if stored out of the refrigerator. In fact, natural products, like food, are often more prone to spoilage than their synthetic petrochemical counterparts.

There are several ways to preserve a product—approximately 15–20 percent ethyl alcohol (grain or SD alcohol) or propylene glycol will do it. Even though these ingredients normally serve other functions, they can preserve the formula at these approximate percentages.[2] Otherwise, some other type of preservation must be used. No preservative is best for all products; in fact, a preservative may be effective in one formula and very ineffective in another formula. Most good chemists use a very low concentration of multiple preservatives to keep the levels of each low, and also to cover a wide range of bacteria, yeasts and molds. Why keep the levels low? Because as concentration increases, some preservatives can irritate sensitive skin.

If it has water (even if it is a part of an extract, infusion, etc.), it must somehow be preserved.

As to the "all natural" claim, keep in mind that "natural" is not in itself a guarantee of safety. There are plenty of highly toxic, irritating, dangerous and even carcinogenic compounds in nature. Focus on "safety," not "natural." I do agree that most of the proven safe, effective ingredients are of natural origin, a fact that leads many of us to focus on natural ingredients. I am a proponent of safe, natural ingredients, but that does not alleviate the work that must be done to insure consumer safety.

---

2   The problem is that at the 15–20 percent level, these two ingredients are not good for our skin.

Most, if not all, of these "all natural" claims are based solely on that supplier's definition of natural, and more than likely, it is not the same as yours.

I like to think the time has arrived for all suppliers to promote products for their safety, performance and ingredients, not for what is *not* in them. A "no preservatives" claim should concern you with the integrity of the manufacturer, and with your own safety.

❀ ❀ ❀

"Contains collagen (or elastin) to reduce sagging skin tissue."

It is true that collagen and elastin are important parts of the skin's muscle tissue system. It is even true that they have great benefit in some skin care formulas as moisturizers and skin conditioners. It is *not* true that an application of collagen to the skin miraculously transforms itself into being supportive tissue under the skin, any more than "hair extract" applied to the skin will grow more hair.

❀ ❀ ❀

"The herbs are absorbed (from the shampoo into the brain) using hair follicles as portals."

It would be nice to scientifically explain why this will not work—the oil in the follicles, the poor absorption of herbs from a shampoo, etc., but only the term "hogwash" comes to mind.

❀ ❀ ❀

"Cleans your hair with pure coconut oil!"

Think about it. When was the last time you tried to clean your hair with oil?

❀ ❀ ❀

"Contains nothing that can give you an allergic reaction such as burning, itching, or rashes, which is caused by chemicals in other products."

Nonsense. It is possible to be allergic to anything. This is ignorance or deception.

❀ ❀ ❀

"Ingredients: Rose Petal Extract, Pure Rose Oil, Quince, Spring Water, Natural Vitamins, Minerals, Salts and Trace Elements from Herbs."

Besides being mostly out of compliance with the labeling law, note that no preservative is listed. One possibility is that the extracts are high in alcohol. If so, that is also required to be on the label. If not, ingredients are missing from the list. The majority of the ingredients listed use improper labeling names.

From a jar label:

"Contains 10% wild yam extract!"

No reason is given why that might be good, but the inference was that this would help women with hormonal problems. There is a species of Mexican yam that is rich in phytoestrogens (*D. composita*), but the one listed in the ingredient list was the wrong one (*D. villosa*). Further, there was no indication of the amount (if any) of the true actives—the sapogenins in wild yam. An extract could be most anything, but "wild yam extract" will not function as implied unless the extract has a high level of these sapogenins. There is no way to tell from this statement. The crucial information is missing. The extract could be completely useless for the intended purpose.

Again, avoid labels and brochures as information sources. They are usually misleading at best.

II Magazine and Newspaper Articles; Other Media

This one is so easy, I almost feel guilty. Almost.

From a natural food industry magazine:

"Propylene glycol: A cheap synthetic humectant made from mineral oil (inferior to vegetable glycerin), propylene glycol is a toxic synthetic used as a carrying agent in herbal extracts."

Gee, do you think the author doesn't like it? Even the price is "cheap." No, it is not made from mineral oil. "Inferior to vegetable glycerin" in what way? (They have substantially different properties.)

It's not only "toxic," it's also "synthetic!" Two magic scare words in one sentence. While she has made it sound similar to toxic waste from the "Acme Chemical Co.," she did neglect to mention that it is approved by the FDA for internal use.

I do not defend propylene glycol as much as I abhor slanted descriptions like this.

Often, when you hear one ingredient praised and another defamed, you find the defamer has some interest in the ingredient he or she praised and not the other.

From the same magazine:

"Alcohol: Alcohol is extremely drying to skin and should be avoided—especially denatured ethyl alcohol, which means that chemicals have been added."

Here is where chemistry gets confusing. Chemists tend to classify many different molecules into groups based on molecular structure. One such class is "alcohols." It is so broad as to include many substances such as the waxy, emollient cetyl and stearyl alcohols, glycerin, vitamin E, poisonous methyl alcohol and the "active" ingredient in beer—ethyl alcohol.

All alcohols are definitely not drying to the skin. In fact, some are moisturizers. Some are essential nutrients or vitamins. Too much *ethyl alcohol* can dry the skin. I suspect this "misdefinition" is just a lack of knowledge, not an intentional slant.

As to the "chemicals . . . added," the author is probably referring to denaturants that are designed to make ethyl alcohol so unpalatable it cannot be consumed mistakenly or used as a source of "drinking" alcohol. There is a wide variety of these denaturants available, depending on the final use of the alcohol (see appendix D).

A second magazine:

"Horsetail Extract: An antioxidant and astringent that regulates and strengthens skin. It is a good source of silicone . . ."

It does not contain silicone (an organic silicon polymer). It does contain *silicon* (not silicone) in the form of silicic acid or silicates.

16

This is *very* different from silicone. While they are close in spelling, they are very different in structure, performance and use.

❀ ❀ ❀

From another magazine:

"Sodium laureth sulfate: Is used as a water softener and in baby shampoos."

Water softener? Completely false. It is a cleanser that *could* be used in baby shampoos, but rarely is.

❀ ❀ ❀

A different magazine:

"Triethanolamine: Organic compound, humectant, emulsifier, pH controlled."

It is *not* an emulsifier by itself, and we've never seen it used as an humectant. pH controlled? Maybe they mean it is used to raise the pH. Organic—yes, in the chemistry sense of the word, not in the "farming" sense of the word.

❀ ❀ ❀

Yet another magazine:

"Sorbitol: Comes from the berries of the mountain ash tree. It inhibits mold and yeast, and replaces glycerin in emulsions, ointments and other cosmetics. It's thick and sticky until diluted."

While sorbitol is found in many berries, it is not commercially available from "mountain ash trees." Yet, a consumer reading this article would believe that is the source. This is purely anecdotal information, passed from article to article. Nor is its main function to inhibit yeast and molds. It is a humectant (moisturizer).

❀ ❀ ❀

Why the errors? Intentional? Anecdotal? Misinformed by the manufacturer? I do not really know.

About three or four years ago, one of the "big three" networks reported that "diethanolamides" in cosmetics were found to cause cancer. ("Cocamide DEA" as it appears on the label, for example.)

I personally called the very reputable group who did the research. I was told a very different set of facts that included:

♦ No, the study did not prove that diethanolamides (DEA) in cosmetics caused cancer. They were, in fact, surprised it was reported as such.

♦ Groups of female and male rats and mice were fed the ingredient in large doses. The mice did not have a higher than normal cancer rate. The rats did.

♦ The control group (not fed the DEA) had a high incidence of cancer also. This is a sign the test may be invalid.

♦ They did no test to simulate use in cosmetics. They were quick to point out that since DEA-type ingredients were primarily used in wash-off products like shampoo and bath gel, there seemed little immediate cause for concern.

♦ The FDA agreed that further testing was necessary and no action was taken, except (quite properly) to call for a retest.

Does DEA cause cancer? If your pet rat eats it, maybe so, maybe not. Could it be a source of cancer? Only maybe at this point. In rinse-off products (shampoos for example) I would not be concerned at this time.

Should *you* be concerned about it? In my opinion, wait for the complete test. If it does concern you, there are plenty of alternatives in the marketplace now.

Do you know how many people were frightened and misled? Probably millions.

Would you be surprised if I told you that a manufacturer who does not use DEA ingredients helped this story along? As I have said before, it is not uncommon for attacks on ingredients to be promoted by someone with an alternative for sale. I request that you ask hard questions before you "buy in" to each new scare on the six o'clock news.

Each time a manufacturer promotes a product by using the phrase "_____ free," the press (and consumers) assumes something dangerous has been removed. This is not always a valid assumption. In some cases it is done solely for the purpose of ensnaring unwary customers.

It is this type of confusion that drives many of us to feel more comfortable with time-tested, natural or naturally-derived ingredients.

Too Good to Be True (But it Is):

A freshman at Eagle Rock Junior High won first prize at the Greater Idaho Falls Science Fair. In his project he urged people to sign a petition demanding strict control or total elimination of the chemical "dihydrogen monoxide."

And for plenty of good reasons, since:

- ◆ It is a factor in excessive sweating and vomiting.
- ◆ It is a major component in acid rain.
- ◆ It can cause severe burns in its gaseous state.
- ◆ Accidental inhalation can kill you.
- ◆ It contributes to erosion.
- ◆ It decreases effectiveness of automobile brakes.
- ◆ It has been found in tumors of terminal cancer patients.

He asked fifty people if they supported a ban of the chemical. Forty-three said yes, six were undecided, and only one knew the chemical was water. The title of his prize-winning project was, "How Gullible Are We?" He was attempting to show how conditioned we have become to alarmists practicing junk science. Frightening, isn't it?

❀　❀　❀

Within the last year, a reporter from one of the "big three" TV networks was reprimanded, and the producer suspended, for falsely reporting that organic foods contained as much or more pesticides than conventional foods. As it turned out, they had not even run the tests before reporting this startling "fact" on national TV.

III   Raw Material Data

This is from a manufacturer's labeling:

"Contains no lauryl sulfates that can damage eyes"

This information may have been extracted from the MSDS sheet that cautions the chemist using *pure* lauryl sulfates to wear eye protection.

The final formulation may have no relationship to this statement. A poorly formulated, high level lauryl sulfate shampoo would probably sting the eyes. Yet all products with sodium lauryl sulfate have been unfairly painted with the same brush.

These kind of statements make it clear the writer completely *ignores* (or doesn't understand) the importance of concentration.

As an example, concentrated hydrochloric acid can immediately burn the skin severely, permanently damage eyes, and even be deadly if ingested. However, it occurs naturally in the stomach, in a much lower concentration, to aid in the digestion of food. In fact, *too little* can be a serious problem.

Is hydrochloric acid "toxic?" Yes. So is selenium, chromium, vitamin A and most other body-essential molecules. Yet, there are safe, even *necessary* and *vital* levels of each. Concentration is very important. Making wild statements about ingredients or their toxicity is irresponsible and muddies the truth.

Toxic on what scale of measurement? As compared to what? Toxic in levels found in cosmetics when applied to the skin? Is toxicity a concern as it is commonly used in cosmetics?

Trace metals are a classic example. Our bodies must have small amounts of chromium, selenium, copper and other trace minerals. They are crucial to overall health and deficiencies can result in disease. There is, however, no argument that they are toxic if consumed in high concentration. Are they "toxic?" It depends on the concentration consumed and *how* they are used.

Estrogen is very beneficial in hormone therapy. There is some evidence that in higher dosages it can be carcinogenic. There is no evidence it has any harmful effect on the skin or body when applied topically. It all depends on how its used and how much is used.

One other thing. Ask the source of this type of "information" another question—"What is the source of your information and may I have a copy of it?" Then, should you ever get it, give it to someone knowledgeable for evaluation.

There are ingredients to be avoided. These irresponsible statements make it more difficult to focus on the real problem ingredients.

IV   Books, Ingredient Dictionaries, Etc.

The following are excerpts taken from popular "ingredient dictionaries":

> *Sodium Lauryl Sulfate: This synthetic substance is used in shampoos for its detergent and foam-building abilities. It causes eye irritations, skin rashes, hair loss, scalp flaking*

similar to dandruff, and allergic reactions. It is frequently disguised in pseudo natural cosmetics with the parenthetic explanation "comes from coconut."

I rarely use sodium lauryl sulfate because too much tends to over-clean. It might be just fine for an oily hair shampoo, or it can be blended with other cleaners and ingredients to provide a more gentle shampoo. The statement above might have you believe that anywhere it appears it is dangerous. That is not true. This is a case of expanding facts and frightening consumers. Probably, not coincidentally, this manufacturer does not use it. It may be prepared from coconut oil or synthetically. It is also approved for use in toothpastes.

In fact, a recent Canadian study suggests sodium lauryl sulfate may inhibit the spread of HIV.

❀ ❀ ❀

"Stearalkonium Chloride: A chemical used in hair conditioners and creams. Causes allergic reactions. Stearalkonium chloride was developed by the fabric industry as a fabric softener, and is a lot cheaper and easier to use in hair conditioning formulas than proteins or herbals, which do help hair health. Toxic."

Facts mixed with partial truths. It is used in hair conditioners and may have been used by the fabric industry for its anti-static electricity features. Note the "causes allergic reactions." This could lead you to believe this is true for everyone. I'm allergic to strawberries, yet I don't wish to have them labeled "causes allergic reactions." Is this an ingredient with a high likelihood to cause a reaction? We can't tell from this description.

"Toxic?" Designed to frighten, not inform. At what level? In any product? Ingested or applied to the skin? Most ingredients have some "toxic" level. Using the word "toxic" by itself is often a tactic designed to frighten you and steer you to a particular manufacturer's product which does not contain that ingredient.

"Cheaper and easier to use?" Why would that be a problem? These are words commonly used to denigrate a material when there is no science behind the argument.

I recommend you avoid manufacturers who rely on scare tactics. Buy products on merit, from someone you trust.

❀ ❀ ❀

And, from the same manufacturer:

"Selenium: A yellowish-brown mineral discovered in the earth's crust in 1807; it is used as a dandruff treatment in shampoos. An excellent treatment for problem scalp; use it in small amounts, as it can irritate the eyes."

Now, when it comes to toxicity, selenium ranks right up near the top on anyone's scale. It is deadly in sufficient concentrations (but safe in extremely low levels). On a one-to-one basis, it is much more "toxic" than stearalkonium chloride. Where is the "toxic" warning here? (Selenium disulfide is used in dandruff treatment shampoos.)

Do you see how a few words added or omitted can alter your opinion?

Do you begin to see how a "slant" could be applied in these "dictionaries?" Concentration is so important.

❀ ❀ ❀

From a popular ingredient dictionary for consumers:

"Glyceryl Caprylate: The monoester of glycerin and caprylic acid."

That tells a chemist something (not much). Don't you feel better now that you know it's a "monoester?" I'll bet it helped you not at all. This is not what a consumer needs to know or probably cares to know. (Remember—this was from a *consumer* dictionary.)

❀ ❀ ❀

From the same dictionary:

"Jojoba Butter: Obtained from jojoba oil."

Not quite. It is sometimes the partially hydrogenated reaction product or the altered isomer (changed molecular shape) of jojoba oil. It is not a component of the oil. Other times it may be a mixture of waxes and jojoba oil.

❀ ❀ ❀

Coco-Betaine: See coconut oil.

Odd, since they are definitely not the same. Nor are they ever used in the same fashion, nor do they have any similar characteristics other than starting with the letters "coco." (This type

of strange cross-reference occurs again and again in this particular dictionary.)

❀ ❀ ❀

*Benzophenone (1–12): A fixative for heavy perfumes and
soaps . . . used in the manufacture of pesticides, antihista-
mines, and hypnotics.*

How would you know that its almost exclusive use in cosmetics
is as a sunscreen?

❀ ❀ ❀

Licorice: Used as coloring in cosmetics . . .

No, it is not, and we cannot find anyone who has ever heard of this
use. (Because licorice *candy* is black, maybe the author assumed
that licorice itself was black—a false assumption.)

❀ ❀ ❀

From the "newly revised edition" of a popular consumer
ingredient dictionary:

Almond oil: See "bitter almond oil."

The author doesn't understand that sweet almond oil (from the
nuts of almond trees, and used in cooking and as a cosmetic emollient) is vastly different from bitter almond oil. When one looks up
"bitter almond oil" in this dictionary, the definition is a jumble of
definitions of bitter almond oil and sweet almond oil. Any consumer reading these explanations would be left thoroughly misinformed. The two ingredients are very different. Bitter almond oil
is the very specific aromatic fraction, used primarily as a fragrance or flavor component and has a higher likelihood of causing
irritation. Sweet almond oil is used as an emollient in skin care
products. It is not surprising that readers of this "ingredient dictionary" would be confused.

V   Price

Our company has developed formulas for, and manufactured for
over 100 different companies.

We once developed an exceptionally good conditioning shampoo for one of them at an incredibly low price. He priced it at a
very low cost. It didn't sell. He doubled the retail price. It then sold

very well. Inexpensive does not always mean inferior. Expensive does not always mean better. Remember:

*"There is no direct relationship
between quality and retail price."*

Most of us believe we are buying more by paying more. In the world of cosmetics that may be true or it may be false. Price alone will not tell us. Use logic and ask questions.

VI   The Sound-Alike Syndrome

Occasionally we are asked why antifreeze is put in skin care formulas. Upon further questioning it is clear that propylene glycol (approved for use in cosmetics, and in fact approved for internal use within limits) has been confused with ethylene glycol.

They do sound similar, and indeed ethylene glycol has been used as an antifreeze and has some toxic effects. But they are not the same ingredient.

Propylene glycol is related to ethylene glycol by the fact that the molecular structure has some similarities. I know what you're thinking—why does it have to be so hard? (Isn't that why you didn't take chemistry?) I reviewed a recent magazine article that said "Propylene glycol is just one molecule away (from ethylene glycol)." Right—and plutonium is just one molecule away from iron. Sometimes it seems the authors just cannot make the story exciting enough without this type of silliness.

Several callers have asked if "urea" (an exceptional moisturizer and skin treatment) is the same as "urine." Happily, we can state for the record, it is not. Nor is it processed from urine.

Avoid drawing conclusions about ingredients that sound similar. You'll find me saying again and again—locate manufacturers on whom you can rely and who will furnish you the information you need. Find out which of them know what they are talking about. Not all do.

VII   Rumors

One of the strangest rumors I have ever heard took place several years ago. Our laboratory 800 number began receiving a large number of calls about an animal-derived ingredient known as "collagen." The question asked again and again was; "Does collagen come from aborted fetuses?" (Were they implying collagen from non-aborted fetuses was okay?)

Of course there is no known commercial source of skin collagen from any human—living or unborn. In attempting to track the rumor we had little success. Was it started by a company not using collagen? Was it a misunderstanding of what collagen is? Did they confuse it with placental extracts? We will probably never know. Regardless, as with most, the rumor soon disappeared.

About three years ago we began receiving calls asking about a new, "dangerous" ingredient called "propyl." Since "propyl" is an adjective and indicates only the length of part of a molecule, it made no sense. We traced the story to a then- popular book about cancer prevention, that hypothesized isopropyl alcohol was involved in the disease. From one page in one book, "propyl" became a blacklisted ingredient. An ingredient that does not exist became very unpopular. Regretfully, any ingredient with "propyl" in the name became needlessly suspect also. Odd how these things have a life of their own.

VIII   Confusion over Internal Use and External Use of Ingredients

Think about alcohol (the drinking variety—ethanol). An excess of ethanol taken internally negatively affects various organs including the brain. It decreases reaction time, slows thinking, can damage our liver, and so forth. Does it do that when applied to the skin? Of course not. It may damage or dry our skin if too much is used on a regular basis, but the overall effect is quite different than if taken internally. So it is with most ingredients.

We see "Contains Vitamin X" emblazoned across bottles and jars, but often there seems to be no explanation of purpose other than the positive connotation of vitamins.

A shampoo claims to have 80 percent aloe. Aloe can be good for you, but how will a very water soluble ingredient like aloe, which will probably end up mostly in our shower drain when we rinse, help our hair?

Another company has recently introduced a line of skin care, claiming it helps you sleep. One of the ingredients is valerian extract, a herb believed to act as a mild sedative when taken internally in fairly substantial dosage. The problem is, we cannot locate a shred of evidence in the scientific world to even suspect that valerian applied externally has similar effects.

Use logic. Ask questions. Don't spend your hard-earned money on such nonsense.

IX   Advertising and Our Desire for a "Quick Fix"

I should know better, but I too listen to those ads for miracle cures.

Nobody does it better than the tabloids. While we have yet to see the headline—"Aliens release Elvis to sell miracle wrinkle cure," we did find the following gem:

"She looks younger than her daughter—overnight!"

Is this what they call "instant gratification?" Twenty years of neglect will not be cured overnight. (Or possibly, her daughter wasn't in such great shape herself and the comparison was correct.)

❀   ❀   ❀

For those of you who are familiar with Dr. Andrew Weil, you have probably heard him speak of "nutritional medicine" and its three parts:

1.   Dietary change   (That will affect the skin greatly.)
2.   Treatment   (Good skin care can help most problems.)
3.   Prevention   (This is what good skin care is all about.)

Notice that finding an "overnight miracle cure" is absent from his list.

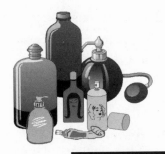

How a Product is Formulated

"If ignorance was bliss, we'd all be a lot happier."
Bumper Sticker (1999)

It is as much an art as it is a science. Sadly, few are really good at it and many lack the understanding of the science behind what they do. That is one of the reasons why you keep switching products, trying to find one that works.

I cannot teach you to be a formulating chemist in these few pages, but I can help you understand what they do. I have broken it down by category to help you follow the formulation. For more detailed information, see the books listed in appendix A, especially references II–A, B & C. These references are very detailed on the subject of formulation of all types of products.

Nor can we cover every type of product in this volume. Those references (II–A, B & C) go into great detail on virtually every category of personal care products.

Cleansers (Shampoos, Bubble Baths, Liquid Soap, etc.)

Here, the formulator's first step is to decide:

- ♦ How much can be spent? This will, by itself, eliminate many ingredients and
- ♦ What type of cleanser it will be? Cream type or foaming?

Foaming Cleansers and Shampoos

These are simply surfactants[1] (cleansing agents) in water. Typically, the water is added first, then the surfactants. They are mixed together and may be heated to complete the solution. If heated, the mixture may be cooled to a temperature where other ingredients can be added. The chemist may add foam boosters, thickeners[2] to increase viscosity, chelating agents,[3] humectants[4] like glycerin, or other surfactants. Conditioning agents, such as protein, are also usually added at this point.

After cooling to a safe temperature (to prevent heat destruction of delicate fragrance oils, herbal extracts, or other actives), these other ingredients are then added. A small amount of solubilizer such as a polysorbate or oleth-20 may be used to help make the fragrance completely soluble. About this time, color and preservatives are added and dissolved in the batch as it is cooled.

Lastly, the pH is adjusted with something like citric acid, then the thickness is increased, if necessary, with salt or some other thickener. The viscosity (thickness) can be reduced in a variety of ways, such as the addition of more water, a small amount of propylene glycol, or by altering the pH. pH alone can have a great effect on the final thickness/viscosity and effectiveness.

Before releasing the batch, the quality control group will complete various tests such as viscosity, pH, batch formula stability, active ingredient analysis, color, odor, density and microbiological purity.

The key items affecting performance are:

♦ The surfactants or blends of surfactants. This generally determines how well it cleans, how much it foams, how "mild" it is, how much it costs and, to a degree, how thick it is. Good chemists usually blend different surfactants to get the best features of each and to reduce the likelihood of irritation.

---

1 See chapter 6 for the definition.
2 Thickeners, such as cellulose gum or its derivatives (an example is Hydroxyethylcellulose), are often the first ingredients dispersed in the water, before the surfactants.
3 See chapter 6 for the definition.
4 See chapter 6 for the definition.

♦ The "actives" that are added. These help the product be more effective, more mild, less irritating, more conditioning, etc. For example, the addition of certain proteins, in sufficient concentration, can help condition or "moisturize" hair or skin. Silicones can add shine and cationics can help prevent "fly-away" hair.

♦ The final pH. This can have a great effect on how well the product performs, or how the skin or hair feels after use. Look for a pH in the 4–6 range, the same pH as skin and hair.

Cream Cleansers

Cream cleansers perform under the theory that "like dissolves like." That is to say that one simple way to remove oily residue is with another oil. (That's why some auto mechanics remove the grease from their hands with oil.)

These products tend to be high oil content emulsions. The process involves at least two separate processing tanks, sometimes three or four.

In tank number one, the water, humectants and some of the other water soluble ingredients are heated to about 150– 180°F. They are mixed until completely dissolved. A thickener may be added first to get it fully dissolved in the water before adding other ingredients.

In tank number two, the oil, oil solubles, waxes and emulsifiers are heated to about the same temperature as tank number one, until everything is melted and homogenous.

Usually, the contents of tank number two are added to tank number one while hot and then mixed well to form an emulsion. (The process can be done in reverse, adding the water solubles into the oils.)

It is then cooled to about 110–130°F to add delicate fragrance oils, herbs, preservatives, active ingredients and colors. The pH is then adjusted and the viscosity checked.

Lastly, the viscosity and color are adjusted. If everything is acceptable, further testing, including testing for microorganism contamination, is completed.

The following are common percentages found in these products:

CLEANSER FORMULATION

Foaming Cleanser		Typical Ingredient Examples
Water	70–90%	usually deionized and sterilized
Surfactants	5–30%	sodium laureth sulfate, cocamidopropyl betaine, disodium laureth sulfosuccinate
Thickeners, Foam Boosters	0–10%	cocamide DEA, lauramide MEA
Humectants	0–5%	glycerin, propylene glycol, sorbitol
Preservatives	0.02–1.0%	parabens, DMDM hydantoin
Actives, Proteins, Conditioners, etc.	0–5%	hydrolyzed proteins, herbal extracts
Fragrance	0.02–1.0%	
Chelating Agent	0.01–0.2%	disodium EDTA, tetrasodium EDTA
Color	Less than 0.1%	FD&C colors, or natural colors
pH Adjusters	0–1%	citric acid, lactic acid, triethanolamine

Cream Cleanser		Typical Ingredient Examples
Water	50–85%	usually deionized and sterilized
Oils	5–35%	fruit or vegetable oils, mineral oil, silicones
Emulsifiers	3–20%	glyceryl stearate, PEG-stearates
Actives	0–5%	herbal extracts, seaweed extract, proteins
Fragrance	0.02–1%	
Preservative	0.02–1%	parabens, diazolidinyl urea, imidazolidinyl urea, phenoxyethanol
Color	Less than 0.1%	FD&C colors or natural color
pH Adjusters	0–1%	citric acid, lactic acid, triethanolamine

Let's wrap this up by looking at an actual ingredient list. We found this list on a very popular mass market shampoo:
The list:

Water (aqua), Sodium Laureth Sulfate, Cocamidopropyl Betaine, Dimethiconol, Silk Protein, Sodium Chloride, Fragrance (parfum), Propylene Glycol, Carbomer, Mica, PPG-9, Guar Hydroxypropyltrimonium Chloride, Tetrasodium EDTA, DMDM Hydantoin, TEA-Dodecylbenzesulfonate, Methenamine, Methylchloroisothiazolinone, Methylisothiazolinone, Titanium Dioxide (CI 77891).

"Decoding" the list; we make the following observations:

(1) The items in parentheses are names used to conform to European labeling laws—ignore them (unless you live there).

(2) **Sodium Laureth Sulfate**—An all-purpose surfactant, cleanser, foamer and thickener. One of the most commonly used surfactants, it is the "primary" ingredient in this shampoo. (More information is in chapter 7.)

(3) **Cocamidopropyl Betaine**—A much milder amphoteric surfactant, probably to provide more foam and cleansing without an increase in irritation potential.

(4) We did not test this formula, but we suspect that everything else is below 1 percent, so the manufacturer can use any order of ingredients he wishes after "cocamidopropyl betaine," or possibly after "dimethiconol." (See chapter 5—"Reading Ingredient Lists.")

(5) **Dimethiconol**—A silicone, to help provide shine and better "comb-out." (This could be more than 1 percent of the formula.)

(6) **Silk Protein**—Usually a conditioning agent

(7) **Sodium Chloride**—Probably used to thicken the product, or as part of another ingredient.

(8) **Fragrance**—Self-explanatory

(9) **Propylene Glycol**—Could be there to adjust (thin) the viscosity, or as a humectant or solvent for another ingredient.

(10) **Carbomer**—A thickener

(11) **Mica**—Contributes to the "pearly" look of this product.

(12) **PPG-9**—I picked this shampoo to point out that even other chemists sometimes are not exactly certain of the function of an ingredient in a particular product. PPG-9 has many uses—surfactant, suspending agent, emulsifier, conditioner, etc.

(13) **Guar Hydroxypropyltrimonium Chloride**—A cationic, quaternary conditioning agent

(14) **Tetrasodium EDTA**—Chelating agent; can also contribute to a higher pH. Also used to increase the effectiveness of preservative systems.

(15) **DMDM Hydantoin**—Preservative

(16) **TEA-Dodecylbenzesulfonate**—Surfactant, solubilizer; may be part of another ingredient because of the low level. Probably part of the dimethiconol pre-mix.

(17) **Methenamine**—Has preservative properties and can contribute to a higher pH.

(18) **Methylchloroisothiazolinone and Methylisothiazolinone**—Preservatives. (Note that there are four or five preservatives in this product; some may perform other functions.)

(19) **Titanium Dioxide**—Provides opacity and white color. In this formula, it may be used to help provide a "pearly" look along with the mica.

Toners

Toners are designed to remove any last traces of cleansers, "tighten" and tone skin, provide astringency, remove excess oil and/or apply an active ingredient. They also help balance the pH of the skin after cleansing, especially if an alkaline cleanser, such as soap, has been used. This extra treatment can help prepare the skin for the application of other products, such as moisturizers.

They are usually simple water, or water and alcohol, solutions. The most common alcohols used are ethanol and isopropanol. The process is usually performed by mixing the ingredients at room temperature or warming them slightly to aid in dissolving some of the more difficult ingredients. The active ingredients and fragrances are added last.

If the alcohol content is low (below about 17 percent) a preservative is needed and it may also be difficult to solubilize the fragrance. Often, you will see a "polysorbate" or "oleth" series ingredient added to obtain a clear solution.

We recommend avoiding the high alcohol content toners as they tend to over-dry the skin. If you see alcohol or witch hazel in alcohol as one of the top two or three ingredients, it is probably not a product for sensible dry skin care. No matter what they claim, toners and astringents do *not* "reduce pore size." You're stuck with what you were given at birth.

If you have dry skin, stick with low-alcohol or alcohol- free toners. This is the perfect product for use of herbals such as aloe, chamomile and sea kelp.

Natural antibacterials used in place of a high alcohol content include camphor, rosemary and grapefruit seed extract.

Creams and Lotions

These are made very much like the cream cleansers previously described in this chapter. The processing is almost identical, but the ingredients are somewhat different.

From a pure formulating standpoint, the difference between creams and lotions is simply their viscosity and oil (or oil soluble) content. Lotions have less oily substances, and are normally less "heavy" or "greasy" feeling. Creams are a more concentrated product, can be more occlusive (but not always) and are thicker, being usually packaged in a jar or tube.

While it is a matter of personal preference, as a general statement, there is less water in a cream and more substance to it.

The higher the oil content (or oil-soluble substances), the higher the amount of emulsifiers you can expect to find in the product.

Gels and Sticks

These are typically water-based products to which thickeners and/or waxes are added to dramatically increase the viscosity. This "gel" characteristic often has little to do with performance and more to do with customer appeal and/or ease of application.

Oils

Usually the simplest of all formulas, oils contain no water (or only a trace).

They range from a single pure oil, to mixtures of oils and esters. Blending different oils is done for several reasons:

- ♦ To achieve a certain "feel" or maximize a certain use, such as a massage oil.
- ♦ To combine the benefits of more than one oil. For example, jojoba oil has a very different composition and effect on the skin than does apricot kernel oil. A blend may suit the intended purpose better than either individual oil.
- ♦ To reduce the negative aspects of a certain oil or oily substance. Natural Vitamin E (tocopherol) is one of our favorite treatments for dry skin. But at the high level (14,000 IU/fluid ounce) we prefer, it is far too sticky to be "cosmetically acceptable." Therefore, we blend it with a lighter oil such as apricot kernel oil to reduce the

sticky feeling. (Examples of other items used to solve this same problem are jojoba oil, squalane, cyclomethicone, isopropyl myristate and isopropyl palmitate.)

♦ To put more ingredients on the label that appeal to customers.

An oil may contain all or part of the following:

Oils	0–100%	
Items added to decrease oiliness	0–50%	(see above)
Solubilizers/Dispersing agents	0–25%	(only needed if it must be dispersed in water, such as a bath oil)
Antioxidants	0.01–0.2%	(to retard rancidity)
Fragrance	0–2%	
Color	0–0.1%	(must be oil-soluble)
Preservative	0–0.2%	(often not used in water-free products)

Note that some oils contain a preservative and others do not.

Generally, without water present, an antibacterial is not necessary. Occasionally, a preservative is added to inhibit the growth of molds in the oil.

The manufacture is usually very simple, requiring simple mixing in very dry equipment. Water, in this case, would be a "contaminant" that could make the finished product cloudy or susceptible to microbial growth.

Sunscreens

Sunscreens are usually creams, lotions, gels or oils, with the active sunscreen ingredient(s) added during processing.

As of this writing, only the following are permitted in the U.S.[5] for the prevention of sunburn:

---

5 See appendix C for Europe and Japan.

	Official Name:	Other Name:
1.	Aminobenzoic acid up to 15 percent[6]	PABA (INCI name) or p-aminobenzoic acid
2.	Avobenzone up to 3 percent	Butyl methoxydibenzoylmethane (INCI name)
3.	Cinoxate up to 3 percent	2-ethoxyethyl-p-methoxycinnamate
4.	Dioxybenzone up to 3 percent	Benzophenone-8 (INCI name)
5.	Homosalate up to 15 percent	Homomenthyl salicylate
6.	Menthyl anthranilate up to 5 percent	Menthyl o-aminobenzoate or Meradimate
7.	Octocrylene up to 10 percent	2-ethylhexyl 2-cyano-3,3 diphenylacrylate
8.	Octyl methoxycinnamate up to 7.5 percent	2-ethylhexyl methoxycinnamate (INCI name) or Octinoxate
9.	Octyl salicylate up to 5 percent	2-ethylhexyl salicylate (INCI name)
10.	Oxybenzone up to 6 percent	Benzophenone-3 (INCI name)
11.	Padimate O up to 8 percent	Octyl dimethyl PABA or ethlyhexyl dimethyl PABA (INCI name)
12.	Phenylbenzimidazole sulfonic acid up to 4 percent	2-phenylbenzimidazole -5-sulfonic acid or Enzilizole
13.	Sulisobenzone up to 10 percent	Benzophenone-4 (INCI name)
14.	Titanium dioxide up to 25 percent	
15.	Trolamine salicylate up to 12 percent	TEA-salicylate (INCI name)
16.	Zinc oxide up to 25 percent	

A last thought about formulating. Consider this possibility: You purchase a cream that touts itself as an "aloe vera," after-sun skin soother. You use it and find that it does not perform as promised. Should you condemn "aloe vera" as an ingredient? Do you tell others that "aloe vera doesn't work?" I would advise against it. Perhaps the amount of aloe vera was too low to be effective. Perhaps it was the wrong type of aloe extract. Perhaps it was the other ingredients inactivating the aloe in a poor formulation. If you must condemn, condemn formulas, not ingredients. All too frequently, too little of a featured ingredient is used, for it to have any positive effect in the product. This is done to get the consumer's attention, and also to keep the price low.

---

6   Maximum level permitted in the U.S. Combinations of sunscreen ingredients must be used to achieve high SPF's.

Find manufacturers upon whom you can rely. You will regularly be disappointed when you purchase products because of a "fad" ingredient emblazoned across the front label. Life is like that. There are those you can trust and those you cannot.

A few years ago, one of the very large mass-market toothpaste manufacturers, introduced a "new" toothpaste, promoted to "Help remove plaque, to help prevent gingivitis." An examination of the new ingredient list revealed only one difference between the new toothpaste and their older version—the addition of red dye. When questioned about how red dye could prevent gingivitis, the answer was that the new brochure inside, helped instruct one about how to prevent gingivitis.

Be skeptical.

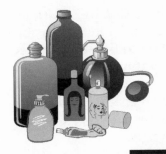

Chapter 4

Sensible Skin Care

"God help those who do not help themselves."
Wilson Mizner (1876–1933)

There are a variety of skin disorders that require a dermatologist's treatment—skin cancers, severe lacerations, extreme cases of acne and so forth.

But the vast majority of us can have healthy, blemish- free, moist-feeling skin if we are willing to put forth minimal effort to learn how to take care of our skin. And we can delay and reduce the onset of wrinkles if we perform some "preventive maintenance." There is no doubt that those who take care of their skin will have fewer wrinkles as they age.

While it is very important to select and use proper skin care, it is no less important to consider the nourishment the skin receives internally.

The skin is the body's largest organ. It can be 5–15 percent of an adult's body weight. It protects us from the environment and from bacterial invasions. It breathes (respires), giving off carbon dioxide. It protects us against dehydration, infection, injuries, foreign substances and temperature extremes.

It helps cool us with perspiration and excretes waste products. Each square centimeter has about 6 million cells, 5,000 sensory points, 100 sweat glands and 15 sebaceous glands. It produces oils, pigments and new cells to regenerate itself. In this same small area, three to five meters of blood vessels and capillaries supply nourishment to the skin.

It is the only organ that can be treated both from the inside and outside. Think of all the supplements promoted for health and for the body's organs. Few of them are designed for the body's largest organ—the skin.

The top (outermost) layers of cells are called the *epidermis*. These are cells that were formed, and have migrated from, the lower (basal) cell layer. During the migration to the surface, they slowly began to flatten, harden and "keratinize," losing their nucleus as they are transformed into the outer physical barrier of the skin, known as the epidermis. The top layers of the epidermis consist of hardened, dead cells known as the *strateum corneum*, which are about 10 percent moisture by weight.

The epidermal cells of the strateum corneum are constantly being shed and replenished by cells from the dermis. This entire process takes about 25–35 days in mature adults. In fact, failure to shed these outer cells properly can be a factor in problems such as dry skin, psoriasis, dandruff and other skin diseases. Properly formulated scrubs and AHAs (alpha hydroxy acids) can alleviate these symptoms if used correctly.

Beneath the epidermis lies the dermis, a highly sensitive, living layer containing nerve endings, fat cells, hair follicles, sweat glands, capillaries and lymph vessels. The dermis is composed of a high percentage of collagen and elastin fibers that provide strength, form, resiliency and firmness to the skin. It is the weakening of these fibers from abuse or oxidation, or the reduction of the amount of these fibers produced as we age, that results in wrinkles and sagging skin.

The subepidermis, below the dermis, is the innermost layer of skin and provides a cushion between the internal bone and muscle, and the rest of the skin. It is a water reservoir that stores fat cells and supports the dermis and epidermis.

Also, as we age, the skin produces less hyaluronic acid and natural oils, which can lead to dryness, irritation, and additional wrinkles.

My own biases will be exposed in this section. I prefer time-tested, safe, edible (if available), natural, non-irritating ingredients where possible. This is usually a much greater challenge and more expensive process than using the petrochemical synthetics. When a superior product can be produced, I prefer to select from the naturally-derived group if a history of use and safety is there. I never hesitate to use preservatives to protect users from potentially dangerous microbial growth. I select combinations with the lowest potential for skin reaction. I am reluctant to use any new synthetics without a long history of safety, because experience has taught me to review and make use of the safety history of each proposed ingredient to screen out potential problems before use.

Natural ingredients have other benefits. There are usually no waste products or toxic materials generated by their preparation. They tend to be multi-functional. They are, of course, renewable if properly harvested. On the downside, they are sometimes scarce, the supply and price can fluctuate greatly and they can have great variation depending on the source. They too can have contaminants, such as pesticides or solvents used in extraction, if a careful, educated selection process is not used.

Internal Treatment

I would be remiss by not stating how important diet is to healthy skin. Most of those items your mom told you to eat— vegetables, fruits, juices, etc., are very good for your skin. A diet rich in anti-oxidants and natural oils (found in most vegetables and fruits) and plenty of water is a good start.

As to supplements, a good multivitamin and mineral (with zinc) is great. Additionally, gamma-linolenic and linoleic acids (GLA) and other essential fatty acids are beneficial to the moisture barrier of the skin, and help maintain a healthy dermis and epidermis. Common sources of the so called "essential fatty acids" are borage oil, cold water fish oils, and evening primrose oil, if you prefer that to a pure supplement. Don't forget how important a variety of antioxidants is in keeping skin looking young and healthy. Antioxidants work together, so a "cocktail" or mixture of them is preferable to any single antioxidant. We prefer micellized liquid supplements because of their superior absorption and the fact that they can pre-solubilize difficult oil-soluble ingredients like beta-carotene and linoleic acid. Your skin requires good nutrition, just like every other organ, but dietary supplements are just that—they are not dietary substitutes. Eat healthy.

It makes sense that skin care is viewed as an external *and* internal treatment program, and it is only natural for a skin care company to have internal supplements to complement their external skin treatments. Experience and test results have shown that liquid micellized treatments are the superior form of these internal treatments. Look for micellized antioxidants like beta carotene, vitamins A, D, and E, linoleic and linolenic acids, and the B vitamins. There are formulas available specifically for skin.

External Treatment

Good skin care is extremely important. The idea that all skin problems are strictly an internal issue has gone on the scrapheap—like the idea that drugs can cure all diseases. In the previous pages, I have shown you how easy it is to "stretch" a claim and damage the credibility of skin care.

But let us not forget some of the wonderful things sensible, effective skin and hair care can do for us.

1. Sunscreens

Sunscreens are a great way to protect your skin from its greatest enemy and prime cause of premature aging/wrinkling—the sun. There is plenty of science here. Just do not be misled into believing that because you don't burn, you suffer no damage. Recent studies indicate that UVA rays still penetrate, and the damage can be cumulative over many years. Sunscreens are there to prevent sunburn. They do not make you invincible. Note that the overall incidence of skin cancer has *increased* since the popularity of sunscreens. There is some evidence that the regular use of broad spectrum (UVA/UVB) sunscreens can reduce the occurrence of moles and freckling in children.[1]

Use sunscreens, reapply them often (no matter what the bottle says), and use them wisely. I would rather have you reapply an SPF-15 every hour or two than stay in the sun for hours with one application of an SPF-30 or 40.

UVB is most potent at the equator and when the sun is directly overhead. UVA is active all day, year round, can penetrate deep into the dermis and can also lead to eye cataracts. Fortunately, melanin in the skin is a fairly efficient absorber of free radicals caused by UVA radiation.

Minimize sun exposure, wear protective clothing, use sunscreens when you must be in the sun, and reapply them often. They will reduce the wrinkles as you get older. Even on a cloudy day, 40–50 percent of the sun's rays reach the earth. Even indoors near a sunny window or outdoors in the shade, we are exposed to UV radiation.

---

1 See bibliography reference no. 45 for more information.

Also remember that a certain amount of UV light is necessary to produce folate, part of the B vitamin complex, and vitamin D3, both of which are essential for good health. Persons with lighter skin color need less exposure than those with darker skin, which contains more melanin to shield out more of the UV light.

2. Antiseptic and Antibacterial Products

These are very important in reducing the spread of disease and helping to prevent infections. Of course, keeping your skin clean is crucial to sensible skin care. Look for a formula with "quats"[2] or natural alternatives, such as grapefruit seed extract, when you need such a product. While we do recommend them for occasional use, it is not a quick solution to preventing every illness. There is even some evidence that overuse of antibacterial products may slowly be weakening our immune system by killing off beneficial germs, and spurring the growth of mutant strains of more resistant bacteria. This has not been proven.

Also a concern, overuse of triclosan and chlorhexidine "may predispose organisms to resistance to therapeutic antibiotics . . ." says a recent American Medical Association report. The opposition claims that it is the over-prescription and misuse of antibiotics that is the real problem. The jury is still out.

Use anti-bacterials, but use safe, natural ingredients, in moderation. Especially when someone else in the household has a communicable illness.

If you are more like myself, and prefer fewer products and "chemicals" in your life, just cleansing frequently with a mild cleanser and warm water will reduce the likelihood of infections. Rinse for at least 20 seconds in cold water to eliminate the warm water environment in which bacteria thrive. Find a gentle cleanser with a safe, natural, antibacterial that you can use regularly. Grapefruit seed extract, lavender oil, tea tree oil and lichen all qualify. (Of course, there must be a sufficient level present to be effective.)

---

2 Many common antiseptics and disinfectants are quaternary ammonium compounds and/or SD alcohol or isopropyl alcohol.

Another benefit of this mild cleansing regimen is the assurance that we are not contributing to the development of "super strains" of bacteria through over-use of chemical antibacterials.

3. Antioxidants

Yes, you can slow down the formation of wrinkles or prevent them. Wonderful things are being discovered about antioxidants and their ability to retard cellular damage and aging—especially for the skin. Now we can understand why people who spend too much time in the sun, or smoke or drink excessively, appear to age faster. These abuses are all prime sources of oxidation reactions.

The theory is this: The body is a complex series of chemical reactions. Some of those reactions, particularly in the cell mitochondria where energy is produced, yield very active, potentially harmful by-products called "free radicals." They attack cell walls, body organs, elastin in the skin and generally are destructive molecules that can age skin faster. (Some free radicals produce elastase, which modifies the elastic fibers and thereby accelerates the aging process of the skin.) There are different types of free radicals and no single antioxidant works well against them all. UV exposure (sunlight) can greatly accelerate the damage. Intelligent formulation calls for a "cocktail" (mixture) of antioxidants. Some antioxidants even regenerate other antioxidants to continue the fight against free radicals.

Examples of some of the better antioxidants are: beta-carotene, green tea extract, ginkgo biloba extract, alpha lipoic acid, glutathione, vitamin E (tocopherol) and vitamin C (ascorbic acid). For those of you who are natural ingredient fans, note that this entire list is comprised of naturally occurring materials.

A recent report from the National Academy of Sciences indicates there is growing evidence that antioxidants contribute to cardiovascular and other disease prevention.

4. Cleansers/Toners

No, it's not breakthrough technology, but there is nothing more important to maintaining healthy skin than proper cleansing. Most people use cleansers that are too harsh and strip most of the protective natural oils from the skin. Find a safe, gentle cleanser and use it regularly. Stay away from toners high in alcohol content.

By way of regular cleansing, via shampoos, hand washes, bath and shower gels, we can easily strip away the skin's protective oils if we use the wrong formulation.[3]

For foaming cleansers, we like those that are based on mild surfactants like cocoamphocarboxyglycinate, coco-betaine, oleyl betaine and TEA-cocoyl glutamate. These are all very mild, naturally derived cleansers. You may notice they do not lather (foam) as well as some of the stronger cleansers. That is not important.

5. Acne Products

Who among us with acne doesn't want to get rid of it or at least alleviate the problem? If you understand that at least three things are necessary for acne, you can better understand how to treat it. The factors (somewhat simplified) that combine to cause acne are; excess oil, blocked pores or hair follicles, and the presence of a bacterium—*Acne vulgaris* in particular.

Treatment may consist of keeping the skin very clean, keeping the pores open and/or the use of antibacterials. While high alcohol products claim to do all three, in reality they can dry the skin, stimulating the oil glands to *increase* the oil flow. We do *not* recommend high alcohol content products.[4]

Cleanse the skin often with a gentle, non-irritating, non-alkaline cleanser. Avoid heavy/oily creams and use as few other products as possible. Look for non–comedogenic products (not likely to cause acne). It is a myth that acne skin is always oily and does not need moisturizing. Look for a non-comedogenic moisturizer specially formulated for acne skin. Tea tree oil is good for use as an antibacterial in these products. Cranberry, camphor and certain other herbals like echinacea or cat's claw also have anti-acne effects. A gentle clay mask can help keep pores open. The only time we would recommend higher alcohol content products is on a direct, localized application to an exist-

---

3   Notice I used the word "formulation," not "ingredient." It is usually the overall formula that dictates mildness (or lack thereof), not any specific ingredient.
4   Except of course, those carrying the label of our favorite winery.

ing pimple or blemish. Salicylic acid[5] is commonly used for its keratolytic[6] effect, and is effectively used up to 2 percent. We are not proponents of the commonly used "Benzoyl Peroxide." In our opinion, it is far too likely to irritate sensitive skin.

6. Burn Treatments

There are a variety of products for minor burns. We recommend those with panthenol, allantoin, echinacea, calendula, aloe, tea tree oil or some other healing agent and/or antibacterial. Always see a doctor for any severe burn, as they can be susceptible to infection.

Honey in high concentration has been used as an antibacterial. Beta-glucan is an excellent aid to healing, as is *fresh* aloe juice.

7. Sore Muscle/Sore Joint Relievers

Capsicum extract (from cayenne pepper—*capsicum frutescens*), whose primary active ingredient is capsaicin, can provide temporary relief to a variety of minor ailments. (Always test it on your skin first—it can produce too much reddening in sensitive individuals.)

Arnica is also used as an external treatment for injuries or pain of this type, as is menthol and methyl salicylate.

8. Massage Products

If you enjoy a massage as much as we do, enough said. Jojoba oil, apricot kernel oil, vitamin E and squalane all function well for this purpose. If petroleum products are acceptable to you, mineral oil is less expensive and has greater "slip" (lubricity).

9. Dandruff Products

You do not have to suffer with this annoying problem anymore. Start by finding a mild shampoo that does not aggravate the problem and use it frequently. Besides the commercial products

---

5   By regulation, 2 percent is the maximum allowable in an OTC (over-the counter) product in the U.S.
6   See "terms" section, chapter 6.

with selenium disulfide or zinc pyrithione, you can find specialty products with tea tree oil and other herbal extracts.

10. Psoriasis/Ecxema Products

There is a variety of products available, but our experience is that each person has to try two or three before finding the one that works for them. Find one that is fragrance-free and free of known irritants and allergens. Remember that claims of "doctor-tested," "hypo-allergenic," etc., have very little legal meaning. They are as good as the company making them.

11. Masks

Besides being a product that makes your face feel wonderful, these products can stimulate circulation, deep clean pores, provide a vehicle for deep moisturizing and temporarily remove fine lines and wrinkles. Masks are also excellent in an acne regimen. Look for clays like hectorite or silt and an antibacterial such as tea tree oil. Other herbals, such as willow bark and cranberry, also possess antibacterial action.

12. Moisturizers

The most common complaint today in skin care is dry skin. Some of our favorite remedies? Hyaluronic acid, natural vitamin E, some seaweed extracts and vitamin E linoleate (tocopheryl linoleate). A study in the *International Journal of Dermatology* in 1994 (vol. 33), demonstrated that the natural hyaluronic acid in our skin (one of its primary moisturizers) was almost depleted by age sixty.

13. Shampoos

Who doesn't use a shampoo these days? Find one that doesn't strip or over-clean your hair. Squeaky clean is not necessarily best. Since we all have slightly different types of hair, find the one that cleans, but doesn't over-clean your hair type. Dry, fly-away hair is caused by over-cleansing and/or lack of conditioners in the product.

14. Hair Loss Products

I have to admit this is often the realm of hucksters, but there is hope for results. Don't plan on waking up to a bushy head of hair after last night's magic hair potion treatment. I am positively convinced that we can slow down or prevent hair loss with proper hair and scalp care, along with proper diet. Start with a gentle shampoo that you can use regularly. Some of the ingredients promoted to assist in keeping the follicles unclogged are polysorbates and jojoba oil. Niacinamide, tocopheryl nicotinate, ivy extract and peppermint are used to stimulate blood circulation on the scalp. Of course a good two- or three-minute massage can accomplish about the same effect. Be sure to massage the scalp, not the hair.

Hair follicles are fed by blood vessels. Therefore complete nourishment through proper diet and good circulation are critical to proper hair health. Healthy hair is the result of all of these plus proper cleansing and as few chemical treatments (color, perms, etc.) as possible. Internally, natural bioflavonoids are often recommended to strengthen capillaries.

15. Skin Lighteners

There are two ways of doing this.

a. **Skin Bleaches**, such as hydroquinone, are fast acting but have a high likelihood of irritation. Further, they are toxic at fairly low levels. Even though they are faster, we recommend you do not use them. (By the way, hydroquinone is banned in several countries, but not in the U.S. where it is allowed only up to 2 percent in OTC drugs.)

b. **Melanin Inhibitors** work much slower, but much safer in our opinion. As skin cells move to the surface of the skin, the melanocytes form melanin (dark pigment) to help protect us from the sun. Melanin inhibitors prevent this melanin from forming, resulting in a very slow lightening of the skin. (It takes about a month for a new, melanin-reduced cell to make the trip to the surface from the lower basal layer.)

Our favorite: magnesium ascorbyl phosphate, a safe, gentle, effective vitamin C derivative. Also used are bearberry extract and licorice root extract.

Ever wanted to lose a few pounds? Somewhere in your mind you know that it really takes more physical exercise, eating better and eating less, along with those appetite suppressants and diet supplements. But . . . those ads for the product that "melts away unwanted pounds while you sleep." . . . are *so* tantalizing. It seems so easy. We *want* to believe it, but of course they really do not help us. Like dieting, we tend to wait until skin problems manifest themselves before we seek a solution. And we are likewise susceptible to those overnight, wrinkle-removing creams we see advertised. For some reason we are skeptical about claims for a pill that will cure a disease overnight . . . but, a magic wrinkle cream? That's different!

Good skin care works. It can improve your skin dramatically, but it functions much better as a preventative than an overnight cure.

The good news is that it is never too late to start.

Just like you can reduce the likelihood of heart attacks and cancer through proper nutrition, so can you reduce the likelihood of premature aging, wrinkling, hair loss and so forth by proper diet and personal care. This is how you do it:

The 10 Steps to Sensible Skin Care

1. Educate yourself.

Stop listening to rumors and stop using magazine articles, biased or uneducated salespeople, and manufacturer's brochures as your source of information. If you do not have time to educate yourself, call several manufacturers. Ask to speak to a chemist and find out how they formulate their products. How do they test them? What is their ingredient selection process? Try their products. Read their brochures. Do they make outlandish claims or do they rely on science and effective products? Stick with two or three manufacturers whom you have "qualified" and with whom you feel comfortable with their formulating philosophy.

Some companies will even let you tour their facilities. Do not expect results from people who are not knowledgeable or honest. If they are using the "kitchen sink" approach, and adding huge numbers of herbs and vitamins to make the label look better, then it is safe to assume they are not reputable. It is most unlikely that anyone could afford to put effective levels of more than two or three herbs in any product.

There is no license requiring you to know what you are doing in order to manufacture skin or hair care products in the U.S. Do not purchase products from companies who make impossible or absurd claims in their ads. Express your frustration with your wallet. If you judge the quality of your products by how well you like the fragrance, you will often be disappointed.

2. Drink plenty of water (more than you do now) and moisturize your skin.

It sounds overly simple, but this alone can make a difference in keeping skin moist and helping carry away waste products. A very small reduction in the skin's water content (about 1 percent), can significantly change the permeability, feel and flexibility of the skin. Healthy skin is about 50 percent water, contributing to softness and flexibility. Too little water can be a factor in dry, flaking or wrinkled skin. Something as simple as a humidifier can help your skin in a dry climate.

Skin constantly loses water through evaporation (especially in low humidity climates) and perspiration. The skin tries to reduce this natural water loss by means of its protective oil barrier, produced by the sebaceous glands. Effectively formulated moisturizers attempt to supplement this natural protection.

Look for ingredients (at proper and useful percentages of course) such as:

♦ **Hyaluronic acid**—It occurs naturally in the skin and is the most powerful "water magnet" available. It is, in our opinion, the best, non-greasy moisturizer and anti-wrinkle ingredient in the world. The natural hyaluronic acid content in our skin declines as we age, until it is nearly gone at age 60.

♦ **Panthenol**—Excellent moisturizer and skin healer.

♦ **Tocopheryl Linoleate**—The superior form of tocopherol (vitamin E), excellent for healing skin and reducing wrinkles.

♦ **Jojoba oil**—Effective skin softener and moisture barrier, similar to the skin's own protective oil barrier.

♦ **Vegetable glycerine and sodium PCA**—Excellent humectants, but can be sticky in sufficient concentration, if not properly formulated.

♦ **Olive oil and olive oil-derived squalene**—Can improve skin dryness if used in sufficient concentration.

♦ **Soya sterol**—Multipurpose, soybean derived emollient, emulsifier and effective moisturizer.

♦ **Dimethicone**—Non-petroleum effective moisture barrier, to prevent moisture loss from the skin.

♦ **Borage oil or Evening Primrose Oil**—Source of gamma linoleic acid to keep the skin healthy.

♦ **Fruit and vegetable oils**—Furnish flexibility and help prevent moisture loss from the skin.

♦ **Beta glucan**—Very effective skin healer, moisturizer and anti-irritant.

♦ **Ceramides**—Duplicate the naturally occurring skin protectants. A common example is **sunflower seed extract**.

♦ **Seaweed extract**—Contains very effective natural, moisturizing polysaccharides.

3. Reduce stress.

Stress does nothing positive for your body and can manifest itself in many ways, including skin problems. Your lifestyle affects your body and your skin. Relaxation therapy is more than a 70s fad. Your body is a fantastic machine. Perform preventative maintenance on a regular basis. Think positively—see the best in life. Get plenty of sleep—it affects your skin.

Relaxed facial muscles tend to form less wrinkles. There is also some evidence that persons who exercise on a regular basis (not in the sun, please) have denser, thicker, stronger skin than do sedentary people.

4. Minimize sun exposure.

This will keep you looking younger, much longer. Use sun-screens (see page 40). Find a light facial moisturizer with an SPF 12–15 that you can use often. (Too high of an SPF can likely irritate sensitive facial skin.) Remember, sun is your number one enemy when it comes to premature aging and wrinkles. Living in Southern California, we often see people who have spent much of their youth in the sun, now looking quite old at about age 35.

Avoid sunlamps. They predominantly emit UVA (less UVB, so you don't burn). UVA is able to penetrate the skin and it is established that UVA contributes strongly to the incidence of skin cancer and damage to DNA. If you don't care about the sun on your skin yet, consider the following fact from Darrell Ringel, M.D., president of the American Academy of Dermatology. As a keynote speaker at a February 4, 2000 academy meeting in Washington D.C. on the subject of sunscreen protection, Dr. Ringel stated that "Every hour, one American dies from skin cancer."

UV radiation can lead to protein "cross-linking," an irreversible process responsible for permanent, deep wrinkling of the skin. One study indicates that UV radiation is responsible for 80–90 percent of perceived aging changes.

Extreme temperatures, wind and pollution also have negative effects on our skin.

5. Keep your skin clean.

Clean it frequently but do *not* over-clean. The target is not "squeaky" clean. Excessive cleansing removes the skin's protective oil barrier and leads to dry skin and increased likelihood of inflammation. Use a gentle apricot seed, soap-free scrub and follow the directions carefully, about once or twice daily. This works especially well if you are taking off make- up at the end of the day. Do not "over-scrub." Also, find a gentle cleanser that you can use regularly to keep your skin clean, but does not dry out your skin or make it feel "tight." Look for gentle cleansers like coco-betaine, cocoamphocarboxyglycinate, decyl polyglucose, sodium cocoyl methyltaurate, TEA-cocoyl glutamate or sodium laureth sulfosuccinate. Cut down on exposure to house/dish cleaning detergents. Get rid of your alkaline soap.

You can identify soaps by: (1) not having a complete ingredient label—they are exempted from the labeling law, or (2) they will have ingredients stating something similar to "fatty acid soap," "tallowate" or "cocoate" of some sort, or list an oil only, when it is clear it is more than just an oil. For example, "made from pure vegetable oil."

Hot baths are to be avoided, or at very least, reduced to an occasional quick soak. These are not good for your skin, as they contribute to the drying of the outer skin layers, especially when bubble baths and other cleansers are in the bath.

6. Avoid fad products until proper research has been done.

(Remember "Phen-Phen™"?) Don't be someone's guinea pig or easy mark. The long-term affect of new ingredients may not be known. I prefer to rely on those that have stood the test of time—proven "natural" ingredients and their derivatives used over at least 20 years without known side effects. It is important to understand that "natural," by itself, is no guarantee of safety. There are plenty of highly toxic, carcinogenic and deadly compounds in nature. Conversely, there are a good number of proven-safe synthetics. Focus on "safety"—not "natural." Find two or three companies who understand this concept. Raving on about how everything natural is good for you demonstrates, at least, a partial lack of understanding.

7. Eat correctly and stop smoking.

Skin is a living organ. Nourish it from the inside as well as the outside. Eat an abundance of *fresh* green, red and yellow vegetables and fruit. If your diet is lacking, supplement with an array of antioxidants such as beta carotene, alpha lipoic acid and selenium (the liquid micellized form is superior), a multivitamin with minerals, and gamma-linolenic and linoleic acids. Make sure you get plenty of vitamins A, D, and E, essential to normal skin health and cell keratinization.

Studies demonstrate that these nutrients are better absorbed in the liquid, micellized form.

Dieting can have a detrimental effect on your skin if the new diet is lacking in skin-essential nutrients. Fruits, vegetables, nuts, whole grains, and cold water fatty fish like salmon, cod and sardines are good for your skin.

Smoking deprives your skin of normal blood flow and stimulates oxidation reactions. In short, it ages your skin faster. Recent studies by British dermatologists suggest that smokers wrinkle prematurely because tobacco activates a gene involved in destroying collagen.

8. Be safe.

Test products before you indulge in them. Many companies do a good job of avoiding irritants and common allergens. That does not mean you will not have an allergic reaction to some ingredient, or a reaction caused by the combination of that product with another product you are using.

Rub in a regular use amount on the inside of your wrist or upper forearm for a day, before a full application. Use a little at first to see how the skin on your face reacts. Never use or continue to use a product that caused a skin reaction.

Good companies (whom you have carefully qualified) in advance, will replace or refund the product via their 800 number if you have a problem. (Some, like ourselves, will even pay the freight to return it.) This is a very important process, because it provides essential information to cosmetic companies about product problems in the marketplace. By returning a product, with information about the problem, you are contributing to that company's base of knowledge about the item.

Never "share" products that you touch, especially makeup. That can transmit bacteria. Never add liquids to change the consistency. That could void the preservative system. Keep all containers, especially make-up, tightly closed when not in use.

Keep all products out of sunlight. Light and heat can degrade preservatives and other ingredients. Throw away or return any product with a drastic change or if an odor develops. Skin care items are all perishable. Preservatives degrade over time and may no longer be effective. Discard all make-up and eye products after three or four months of use. Avoid inhaling aerosol spray products. They may cause lung damage if inhaled regularly. If you get an eye infection, throw away all eye products you were using. It is not worth the risk. Always use a new disposable applicator for testing products at the sales counter.

9. Find and use great skin care.

Limit it to what your skin needs. *More products are not necessarily better, and, in fact, can increase the likelihood of a skin reaction.* Do not change products too often—find one that works and stick with it. Our recommendations:

A. A gentle, moisturizing cream scrub—once or twice a day, following directions carefully. Exfoliation can remove dry patches of dead skin cells and reduce dry skin. There are many types available, ranging from very hard pumice and salt crystal types, to softer jojoba wax bead, polyethylene and almond meal scrubs. The softer the particle, the less effective they are, and our studies indicate that apricot seeds provide the right combination of effectiveness and gentleness, if properly formulated.

B. A gentle cleanser—as often as feasible for you during the entire day. If your skin feels dry and taut after cleansing, find a better one. Gentle surfactants like TEA cocoyl glutamate, decyl polyglucose, sodium methyl cocoyltaurate and sulfosuccinates are excellent. Always rinse very well, with warm to cool water, after each cleansing.

C. A non-drying toner—to follow the cleanser, preferably with antibacterial properties but *not* high in alcohol. This also helps prepare your skin for further treatment. Use the toner to remove any last traces of cleanser and to begin the moisturizing process. If you are a fan of aloe vera, this is the perfect application. Camphor, tea tree oil and calendula are excellent natural antibacterial for these products. Ginseng, beta glucan and licorice root are skin soothers often used in these formulas. Niacin is a great circulation stimulator.

D. An all-purpose, light SPF 12–15 facial moisturizer, light enough to be worn under make-up (preferably with antioxidants). Moisture and humectants can make a real difference in your skin. Use a rich, soothing body lotion right after every bath or shower. Do not *allow* your skin to feel dry. Moisturize frequently. When selecting an SPF, remember more is not necessarily better. The higher the SPF, the greater the likelihood of irritation on the face. Stick with a 12–15, which will be increased by the physical UV blocking of make-up. If you do not wear make-up, or for areas of the body other than the face, reapply every hour or two.

E.   An antioxidant rich cream for day or night time use. This is the place for the oils and/or occlusive products if you like them. Nourish your skin at night. Look for a mixture of antioxidants like beta carotene, selenium, vitamins A, E, and C, ginkgo biloba and green tea. Apricot kernel oil, soya sterols, lipoic acid, lactic acid, chamomile and tocopheryl linoleate are all excellent treatments. When it comes to Vitamin E (tocopherol), the pure oil is superior, but somewhat sticky. Use about 14,000 I.U. per ounce if it's not too oily for you. ("d l-alpha" indicates synthetic tocopherol. "d-alpha" indicates natural tocopherol, a more active form.)

F.   A clay mask with the ability to deep-clean pores and keep them unblocked—about 2–3 times a week. Hectorite and silt are two very effective clays.

G.   For very dry spots, use an intensive moisturizer with a high d-alpha tocopherol, d-alpha tocopheryl acetate, or tocopheryl linoleate content. Vegetable glycerin, fruit and vegetable oils, soya sterols, squalane, seaweed and/or azulene are examples of intensive moisturizers (if used in a sufficiently high concentration).

H.   Use special products only as needed:

(1)   Acne formulas (see page 43)

(2)   Anti-wrinkle treatments and peels (look for hyaluronic acid, lactic acid, glycolic acid, papaya enzyme peels, retinol and antioxidants).

(3)   Psoriasis, ecxema, rash treatments (look for high concentrations of vitamin E, D, tocopheryl linoleate and vitamin A).

(4)   "Dark circle" removers (azulene, live yeast cell extract, ginseng, green tea and cypress extracts are effective in sufficient concentration).

(5)   Sunscreens—SPF 10 and above in the sun.

I.   Look for a pH between 4.0–6.0 for your regular use, leave-on products. Special-use items such as alpha hydroxy acids or masks may deviate from this recommended range. Healthy skin has a natural pH within these limits to ward off bacteria and to help keep skin soft and supple. This is known as the skin's "acid mantle." Harsh cleansers or alkaline products (higher pH) can disrupt this protection, resulting in dry skin, irritation or a thickening of the skin. Avoid soap!

J. Contrary to the "advertising and marketing scientists," oily, dry and normal skin do not necessarily need different products. Great products generally work for everyone. The exceptions might be toners and moisturizers.

K. Find a company that understands the formulation of *low-irritation* products. Some of the basics are:

(1) Removing commonly known allergens and irritants, neutralizing them, or reducing them to a level at which they become innocuous.

For example, nickel, a known problem, can be chelated ("neutralized") by use of various EDTA compounds.

There are ingredients that act as anti-irritants. Examples are: kola nut extract, oat flour and licorice root.

(2) Selection of high purity, high quality raw materials with no or few contaminants, especially those with the potential to be an allergen. For example, a recent study showed that eight of twenty-two brands of Korean ginseng contain high levels of pesticides or lead. This is not a business for companies that do not or cannot do their homework.

(3) The product must be properly preserved. The preservatives must be carefully selected and be at so low a level as to be non-irritating. Antioxidants must be used to prevent product degradation if natural oils are present, otherwise they will turn rancid, just as do the cooking oils you use at home.

(4) High levels of solvents and strong cleansers should be avoided as they encourage skin penetration and damage the skin's lipid barriers, increasing the penetration of other ingredients. Examples are "ethanol"

and "isopropanol." The same ingredient in two differing formulas can have a very different potential to irritate the skin, depending on the level used and the other ingredients.

(5) Recognizing that occlusive type formulas (heavy, skin blocking types; see page 87) can have beneficial effects, but can also inadvertently increase penetration of some ingredients by blocking the normal skin functions.

Absorption into the skin is affected by (1) the integrity of the skin barrier, (2) the physical/chemical properties of the substance, (3) occlusiveness, (4) site of application (regional differences exist in skin thickness), (5) the solvents and/or emulsifiers in the product, (6) the amount applied, (7) temperature, (8) personal metabolism, (9) age (infants, for example, are more likely to have a response), and (10) pH.

(6) Careful selection of the cleansing agents and the level used, to avoid over-cleaning the skin and damaging the skin's protective lipid barrier. High levels of some anionic cleansers should be avoided.

(7) Using as few ingredients as necessary. Loading up the formula to make it look good is not in your best interest. It can increase the chance of irritation.

10. Ask questions.

Use logic. Think prevention. Believe in miracles from God, not overnight wrinkle-removing creams.

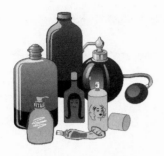

Chapter 5

Reading Ingredient Lists and Labels (If You Must)

"We don't know a millionth of one percent about anything." Thomas Alva Edison (1847–1931)

In the U.S., the labeling law is very clear (but occasionally not followed). Ingredients must be listed on the label per the following criteria:

1. By the Proper Designated Name

I won't bore you with the entire section of law. Just understand that very little latitude is given in how the name must appear. Here are a few examples of common names, which must be changed for proper listing.

Trade or common names:	Correct listing on the label: (INCI[1] name)
Salt or Sea Salt	Sodium Chloride
Vitamin C	Ascorbic Acid
Vitamin A Palmitate	Retinyl Palmitate
Alpha Hydroxy Acids	Lactic Acid, Glycolic Acid, etc.
Aloe Vera	Aloe Barbadensis Gel
Gotu Kola Extract	Hydrocotyl Extract
Animal Keratin	Keratin or Hydrolyzed Keratin
Bicarbonate of Soda	Sodium Bicarbonate

---

1   International Nomenclature of Cosmetic Ingredients.

Trade or common names:	Correct listing on the label: (INCI name)
Borax	Sodium Borate
Cayenne Pepper	Capsicum Frutescens or Capsaicin
Corn Sugar Gum	Xanthan Gum
Vitamin E	Tocopherol
Distilled Water or Spring Water	Water
Vitamin D	Cholecalciferol
Gum Arabic	Acacia Senegal

As you can see, this law (The Fair Packaging and Labeling Act) is not always consumer friendly when it comes to deciphering names, and we haven't even covered the names that are undecipherable whether it is a common or INCI name. Can you possibly guess what any of the following might be?

PEG-53 Butyl Ether	DMDM Hydantoin
PEG-4 Stearate Phosphate	Methyl Gluceth-20
Nonoxynol-20	Quaternium-18
Dimethicone Copolyol	Ozokerite

Of course not. In fact, about half the ingredients in a typical list may be undecipherable without getting information from a competent source.

As I cautioned you earlier, do not fall into a "syllable safety" evaluation. Those who subscribe to this notion feel that the more syllables in the name, the more dangerous it must be—a completely false assumption. Short names do not guarantee safety. Ever hear of dioxin? DDT? Ricin? (Ricin is a very deadly poison extracted from the castor bean plant.)

How about "Codecarboxylase?" Lots of syllables and it sounds intimidating, but it is a very safe form of vitamin B_6. Thiamine Hydrochloride? Vitamin B_1. If I really wanted to scare those easily frightened by word length, how about the chemical name for ascorbic acid or vitamin C? L-3-ketothreohexuronic acid. That almost scares *me*. Glycerin? 1,2,3, propanetriol. As you can see, long names do not have anything to do with safety. Occasionally, I will begin a seminar by asking if anyone can identify the following: 1,8-dihydroxy-3-hydroxymethyl-10-(6- hydroxymethyl-3,4,5-tri-hydroxy-2-pryanyl) anthrone. Just when they begin to suspect it is a toxic, carcinogenic and dangerous waste product, I advise them it is one of the main components of the aloe vera plant—aloin. It's easy to be fooled by long names.

2. In Descending Order of Predominance

The ingredients must be listed in descending order of predominance, highest weight percentage is listed first, followed by all ingredients in descending order including all of those present at 1 percent or more. That is why "water" usually is the first ingredient, unless it is disguised as an "infusion" or "extract" solvent.

What about ingredients below 1 percent? They are permitted in a list (after those at 1.0 percent or higher), in any order the company wants, and are often jumbled not to deceive customers, but to confuse competitors. All colorants must be listed last, and must be FDA approved colors. (Colors are the only pre-approved ingredients in the U.S.)

3. Exceptions to the Law

a. Trade secrets (which must be approved in advance by the FDA) may be listed solely as " . . . and other ingredients" if approved. (They rarely are approved.)

b. Manufacturing aids need not be listed. This is somewhat of a gray area. For example, ingredients used to reduce foam or to aid in filtering during processing are apparently exempted.

c. Products for use *only* in salons and by beauticians, *and* labeled "For Professional Use Only" are exempted from ingredient labeling.

What happens if one uses a plant extract that is 1 percent plant material and 99 percent solvent (water, glycerin, alcohol, etc.)? One is supposed to list the solvent and the plant. It is common to see it placed in the list where the total percent would fit. For example if a formula contained 7 percent of this 1 percent extract it is often placed where a 7 percent (concentrated) ingredient would fit, not where a .07 percent (1 percent of 7 percent) extract would go in the list. Is that within the regulations? It's somewhat of a gray area, but I could guess what the FDA would say.

59

I can imagine you have had enough of the rules. Suffice it to say, the letter size, placement of the ingredient list on the container, net contents declaration, and company name information are also prescribed by law.[2] Now, how do you get useful information from the list?

Use this thought process to scan the ingredient list:

1. First, look for items to which you know you are allergic (if any) or do not want to use for safety reasons. Learn their label names so you can quickly identify them. If you do not know how they appear on a proper ingredient list—call one of the sources I listed and find out.

2. What are the "active" ingredients? Is there any clue on the literature or label? If it says "panthenol to heal skin" and panthenol is number 17 on a list of 20 ingredients, you can assume there is not a large amount in the product.

    Perhaps a call to the company is warranted for an explanation. You have to be careful to a degree, because certain actives (like vitamin A acid, for example, require a considerably lower percentage than an active like panthenol or collagen).

    The following are proper concentrations for effectiveness of some of the more common active ingredients:

Jojoba Oil	1–10%	Hyaluronic Acid	0.1–0.5%
Proteins	0.5–5%	Alpha Hydroxy Acids	1.0–12%
Vitamin E	0.2–3%	Panthenol	1.0–5%
Allantoin	0.1–0.2%	Vitamin A	0.01–0.5%
Ascorbic Acid	0.5–10%	Beta-Carotene	Look for a yellow color in the product
Tea Tree Oil	0.5–10%	Honey	5–20%
Collagen	2–10%		

---

2 Regrettably, many smaller companies are often in violation of the complex regulations, simply because they do not understand them completely.

3. The colorants are always last. If you object to artificial colors, look there for such things as FD&C Yellow 5,[3] D&C Green 5,[4] Blue 1, etc.

4. Want unscented products? Look for the word "fragrance" or any of the aromatic oils such as peppermint, ylang-ylang, orange, lemon, sage, etc. Products containing these are not "unscented," regardless of what the label might say. Use your nose to verify this.

   All ingredients used as fragrances may be listed separately, or together as "fragrance." This is not a signal as to natural or synthetic origin. Many natural oil users will list all the oils separately instead of using the term "fragrance" in the ingredient list. Sometimes it is impractical to list all of the oils in a sophisticated, complex fragrance as there is not enough space on the label. There can be as many as 200 ingredients in such a fragrance blend.

5. Is the ingredient just there for "show?" Sad to say, but in my opinion most herbal extracts are added not for their efficiency, but for their appeal to the consumer. Usually (not always), it requires 2–20 percent of an herbal extract to make a real difference in a product. Check out where the herbs and other actives appear in the ingredient list. It is my estimate that about 95 percent of all herbals are added for ingredient "show," not function. In many cases it is because the manufacturer does not understand or believe in herbal effectiveness. I am certain some of them are very effective at *sufficient level*, with the *correct extract*. Examples are capsicum, aloe, tea tree oil, azulene (from chamomile), licorice, ginseng, seaweed and gingko biloba.

   Be especially wary of ingredient lists containing more than two or three herbals. It is usually a signal that not enough of any one herbal is present in sufficient concentration. From a formulation effectiveness standpoint, it just doesn't make sense, and it is likely they are there only to

---

3 "FD&C" means it is FDA-approved for use in foods, drugs and cosmetics.
4 "D&C" means it is FDA-approved for use only in drugs and cosmetics. Why is it OK for drugs but not for foods? Because it is. I don't necessarily agree with all regulatory logic. It has something to do with the risk factor and amount consumed in foods versus drugs.

dazzle the unsuspecting consumer. From a price perspective it is almost impossible to have all of them at effective levels.

6. Use the attached ingredient dictionary to look up those ingredients with which you are unfamiliar. The dictionary is not complete (there are thousands of ingredients available) but we tried to cover many of the most commonly used materials. Future editions will add to this list. Keep in mind that a good formulation can often overcome some of the negatives.

7. Few things confuse customers more than preservatives. As I said earlier, if water is present, preservatives are mandatory for your own safety (unless you are willing to keep your products frozen). Do not believe these "preservative-free" claims if water is present, whether it be listed as water, an aqueous herbal extract or infusion, or otherwise. In fact, use that as a warning about other product claims the company makes. Some of the more common preservatives are:

Methylparaben
Ethylparaben
Imidiazolidinyl Urea
    (Germall™)
Grapefruit Seed Extract
Potassium Sorbate
SD Alcohol
Quaternium 15 (Dowicil™)
Triclocarban
EDTA
Boric Acid
Glutaraldehyde
DMDM Hydantoin
2-Bromo-2 Nitropropane-1,
    3 Diol
Methylchloroisothiazolinone
Triclosan
Butylparaben
Cresol
Phenol

Propylparaben
Diazolidinyl Urea
Phenoxyethanol
Sodium Hydroxymethyl-
    glycinate
Sorbic Acid
Propylene Glycol
Chloroxylenol
Methylisothiazolinone
Sodium Dehydroacetate
Formaldehyde
O-Phenylphenol
Chlorphenesin
Methenamine
Benzalkonium Chloride
Benzyl Alcohol
Benzethonium Chloride
Chlorbutanol
Iodopropynl Butylcarbamate

8. We will list some ingredients to avoid in the ingredient dictionary. Besides not knowing the use percentage, another problem with trying to evaluate safety from ingredient lists is that by-products, contaminants, and minor "ingredients of ingredients," do not have to be listed. For example, the

consumer has no way of knowing if the mineral oil on the label is 100 percent pure, or contains smaller amounts of other, more dangerous hydrocarbons. Neither can you tell if the herbal extract on the label was grown and harvested organically, or contains trace amounts of pesticides. Nor can you tell how much (if any) free "DEA" is still present in the "Lauramide DEA" on the label. We must rely on our product suppliers. Investigate and qualify them.

As an example of the unknowns that do not appear on labels, consider the case of the different mushroom extracts. Because mushrooms can be grown under very different conditions, and because they tend to absorb toxins, the wrong extract can contain ingredients unfit for human products. Further, the age at which they are picked can be crucial to the active ingredient content. Unless a formulator has done his/her ingredient research in a very diligent fashion, the extract may at best be ineffective, at worst potentially dangerous, and they would all appear on the label as the same extract. It is not an uncommon practice for a manufacturer to completely rely on the integrity of his supplier—a potentially dangerous method of raw material selection.

Because this section is so very important, I want to restate it. *You are completely relying on the integrity and investigative thoroughness of the manufacturers when it comes to minor ingredients of an ingredient.* The minor ingredients do not have to be listed on the label.

9. Unless you are a chemist, there is little more you can do except:

    a. Refer to the dictionary in this book.

    b. Call the "800" number on the container—always ask for a chemist in the lab—*not* the sales department. Chemists are usually more direct and factual than sales people,[5] simply because they know more about the ingredients and less about sales.

    c. Build personal confidence in two or three companies upon whom you can rely. Support their integrity by

---

5 Except our own, of course.

using their products, and your skin will improve because of it.

There are volumes available about cosmetics, but to our knowledge, no proper ingredient dictionary exists for all of the ingredients. If nothing else, we hope this book will enable you to ask the right questions and provide the names of references and resources for further investigation.

Favorite Words of Copy Writers for Cosmetic Products

If it is your intention to decipher diligently the claims that appear on cosmetic labels or literature, you should become more aware of the following common "hedge" words:

"Helps"

This can mean most anything. Usually it refers to the fact that the product does *not* perform the intended function completely. Could also be used as a "hedge" word to avoid making a drug claim that involves changing the physiology of the skin, as in, "Helps reduce dry skin," a cosmetic claim, versus "Cures dry skin," a drug claim.

"Reduces"

Usually indicates the product does not completely alleviate the problem it is intended to solve.

"Firming"

Intended to imply that the skin will be more taut (or less "sagging"). A purposefully vague term that has positive connotations.

"Brighter," "glowing," " radiant," etc.

Vague terms that mean little. Could indicate that circulation in the skin has been increased, resulting in a more rosy (reddish) appearance.

"Younger-looking," "Healthy-looking," etc.

While this seems clear enough, little can be concluded because this favorite term is entirely subjective and has no legal definition. Since it is impossible to make skin "younger" and since "healthy" implies to the FDA that a disease has been cured, the qualifier "looking" is usually added.

"Effective"

Usually not tied to any direct claim, leaving the reader to ask—"Effective at what?"

"Almost"

Translate as "Not quite what it is claimed to be."

Read claims of effectiveness carefully. If the claims are too good to be true, they probably are. If they are hedged by the words above, be a bit skeptical. Another advantage of qualifying a company with a good return policy, is that you can simply return the product if it does not perform to your satisfaction.

Good skin care works, but it will usually involve a little effort on your part, and rarely does it come from companies making outrageous and unsubstantiated claims. Do you really want to do business with a company that is obviously not telling you the complete truth?

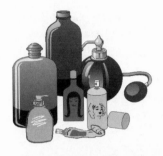

Chapter 6

Dictionary of Terms Used in Cosmetics

Abrasive: Typically, irregularly shaped, fine or coarse solids. Usually natural in origin, either mineral (pumice, chalk, phosphates, diatomaceous earth) or vegetable (almond meal, apricot kernels, walnut shells, oatmeal, jojoba wax, corn starch), abrasives are used in cosmetics to remove dead skin cells, callus, dirt, debris or material on teeth. Not all abrasives are created equal. More rounded and/or softer particles are less abrasive, but also less effective.

There are those who claim scrubs are dangerous to the skin. They are not harmful if properly formulated, and can be quite beneficial as part of a serious skin care program. This process, termed "exfoliation," removes dead skin cells and debris from the skin, stimulates circulation and the growth of new cells, and helps keep pores unclogged.

Absorbant/Adsorbent: Solids (usually) with large surface area which can attract substances from another medium. May be used in manufacturing process, i.e., to remove hazy, fine particles from a product; or as the function of the product, i.e. kaolin or clay in masks, rice starch to absorb oils, etc. By definition, absorption is a process where the material being absorbed is taken into the absorbing medium. Adsorption is in the attachment of a substance to the surface of the adsorbing material.

Acid: A large group of different ingredients so named for their acidic pH (less than 7). It includes the mineral acids—sulfuric, hydrochloric, nitric and the like.

More important to personal care, it also includes the weaker organic acids such as ascorbic, tartaric, glycolic, lactic, citric, etc.

The strength of an acid is related to the pH of the solution. The lower the pH, the more acidic it is. As the pH increases, the acids become more neutralized. The pH of skin is slightly acidic.

Generally, the pH of skin and hair is between 4.0 and 6.0. Very alkaline pHs (8 and above) such as those found in soap, tend to cause a dry, tight feeling in skin, and are drying to the hair. (Also see: "pH"; "Alkaline")

Acrylates: Salt or esters of acrylic acid which are polymerized (see Polymer) to form products used as thickening agents, hair fixatives, skin protectants and nail polishes. While the unpolymerized materials are strong irritants, the polymers generally are much safer and less likely to cause irritation.

AHA: (See "Alpha Hydroxy Acids")

Alcohol: The term "Alcohol" is the name given to a very large group of very different ingredients ranging from nutrients like panthenol, moisturizers and emulsifiers like cetyl and stearyl alcohol, to volatile alcohols used in perfumes and hair sprays (ethanol), to poisonous methyl alcohol. No safety (or lack thereof) can be inferred from the general term "alcohol." Each alcohol must be reviewed on its own and in the concentration present.

The term "Alcohol" is often interpreted by laypersons to mean ethyl alcohol (AKA *ethanol*, grain, or drinking alcohol) or isopropyl alcohol (AKA *isopropanol* or rubbing alcohol). These two alcohols are relatively powerful solvents.

In general, high concentrations of ethanol (SD alcohol) or isopropyl alcohol can be very drying to the skin, and increase penetration, raising the likelihood of irritation. Ethanol is used in perfumes, colognes and in hair sprays to solubilize ingredients and help the formula "spray" well and dry quickly.

Vitamin E, glycerin, and panthenol are also alcohols and quite beneficial to skin.

Aerosol: A product dispersed from a sealed container by means of a pressurized gas. Many hairsprays are aerosols.

Alkaline: Solutions having a pH above 7.0. Most detergents and all soaps are alkaline. Alkaline cosmetics or alkaline soaps can upset the skin's natural pH balance. Excess alkalinity dries the skin and reduces its resistance to irritation and infection. It can also make hair brittle, dull and hard to manage.

Soaps, by their very nature, are alkaline. This helps account for the dry, tight feeling they often contribute to the skin. For this reason, other ingredients are often added to the soap in an attempt to overcome this problem.

Alkanolamide: A type of alcohol, a special group of amides used in cosmetic formulation. Alkanolamides are used as surfactants, foam boosters, viscosity enhancers and are occasionally used as emulsifiers. They are the product of the reaction between fatty acids and alkanolamines.

The most commonly used is cocamide DEA.

Alkanolamine: A special group of substances formed from amines which do not have the volatility or strong odor characteristic of amines. The most widely used alkanolamines are mono-, di-, and tri-ethanolamines, which are frequently abbreviated as MEA, DEA and TEA. Widely used as raw materials in the production of cosmetic ingredients, alkanolamines are used directly to neutralize various acids and to adjust the pH of cosmetic products. (Also see: "Alkanolamide")

Allergen: Any substance which, when it comes into contact with body tissue (by skin absorption, ingestion, or inhalation), causes a specific reaction within the bloodstream. An individual's (allergic) response to an allergen can be inherited. Allergens are typically proteins (wool, milk, pollen, etc.). Allergens can be found in many plant products, some are metals (such as nickel), and a few are organic compounds.

It requires two exposures to develop an allergic response. Response varies from individual to individual and sensitivity may develop over time.

It's actually more complicated at times because of the problem of "compound allergens." Evidence is available to suggest that ingredients of a preparation or ingredients from more than one source can interact to form a new allergen. For example, EDTA, hydrocortisone or 2 percent miconazole nitrate separately do not normally induce an allergic reaction. However, in combination they can produce a compound allergic reaction.[1]

Skin rashes attributed to cosmetics are often, in reality, caused by dress or sheet fabrics, jewelry or other causes or multiple causes.

The most common cosmetic complaints are from perms, deodorants, and other products normally allowed to remain on sensitive parts of the body.

Alpha Hydroxy Acids (a-hydroxy acids): The most commonly used are glycolic and lactic. In low concentration and acidic pH, they are moisturizers. In higher concentrations and more acidic pH (below about 5), they are exfoliants. They work by loosening the material that holds surface skin cells together. High concentrations above approximately 8 percent can over-exfoliate, peel and make skin red if not properly formulated. AHA's can also improve the natural hyaluronic acid content of the skin and help reduce dark spots. Commonly derived from natural sources such as sugar cane (glycolic) or citrus fruits.

---

1   Bibliography reference no. 5.

It is important to note that pH and concentration are both determining factors. The same concentration at pH 6.0 is much less effective than that at pH 4.0. Overuse can cause "skin fatigue," meaning that the skin is temporarily over-treated, sensitized and no longer receptive to improvement. The effect is reversible after discontinuing use for a few weeks. In high concentration, use them sparingly.

Note that for skin care purposes, studies show little performance difference between AHAs and the closely related organic acids, BHAs (beta hydroxy acids).

Amide: A nitrogen based molecule derived from, or related to, ammonia. Amides are commonly formed from the reaction between a fatty acid and an amine. Amides are used as moisturizers, preservatives, surfactants, and foaming agents.

Amine: Organic compounds built upon ammonia (NH2) are amines. Amines are the building block for quaternary ammonium compounds, alkanolamines and amino acids. Amines that do not carry additional function groupings usually have unpleasant odors and are, therefore, not widely used in cosmetics.

Amino Acids: The building blocks of proteins, some of which (essential amino acids) must be supplied externally to support body's growth. Necessary internally for the growth of hair, skin, and nails as well as all connective tissue and genetic material. Generally, amino acids are weak acids which behave differently in products, depending on the pH of the solution. At intermediate pH, near neutrality, the amino group is amphoteric. Amino acids are used in personal care products as skin and hair conditioners.

Amino acids linked together are named polypeptides. As those groups increase in molecular length, they are called proteins. (Also see: "Protein")

Amphoteric: Having the ability to act either as an acid or a base. Proteins and amino acids are amphoteric, containing both a base group and an acid group (wool is an amphoteric which can absorb dyes which are acidic or basic). Amphoteric surfactants can perform in hard or soft water, which may be alkaline or acid, and still remain effective and gentle. In acidic solution they become positively charged, in an alkaline environment they have a net negative charge.

Amphoteric cleansers are particularly known for their *mildness to skin and hair*. Examples are disodium lauroamphodiacetate, cocoamphocarboxyglycinate or sodium lauriminodipropionate.

Anionic Surfactant: Characterized by a negative charge on the hydrophillic (water soluble) portion of the molecule. This group includes some of the stronger cleansers.

Alkyl sulfates are the most widely used, made up of a long chain hydrocarbon with a sulfate group on one end.

Antioxidant: An ingredient added to natural fats and oils which retards oxidation and rancidity. Typical examples are vitamin E, BHA, BHT. (Rancid oils and fats can act as skin irritants, and have an unpleasant odor.)

A second, more popular group, is used to neutralize excess toxic "free radicals"[2] in or on the body which are believed to contribute to the aging process if left un-neutralized. Excess free radicals can be caused by sun exposure, pollution, fried foods, smoking, excessive alcohol, stress, physical exercise, and certain chemicals. The body normally produces certain amounts of free radicals, the danger being in over-production. If the balance is disrupted, aging may be accelerated.

Much of the current research into anti-aging focuses on free radicals and antioxidants, or natural products that contain antioxidants. Examples are: ascorbic acid, ginkgo biloba extract, beta carotene, tocopherol, coenzyme Q-10, lipoic acid, glutathione and green tea extract. Antioxidants generally interact with one another and this antioxidant network is important to the overall bodily defense against free radical damage and aging. For example, coenzyme Q-10 can regenerate vitamin E in the body.

Antiperspirant: A product which, when applied under the arm or on other skin, will reduce perspiration at that site. All antiperspirants are over-the-counter (OTC) drugs in the U.S. and are regulated by the FDA. All antiperspirants contain aluminum or zirconium salts. Deodorants are not regulated as drugs and generally do not contain aluminum antiperspirant ingredients.

Because they block the natural perspiration process, it is argued that they contribute to toxin build-up. While aluminum has been implicated in Alzheimer's disease, we have not seen definite proof that it is a cause. Studies are underway at this time.

Antiseptic: Ingredients capable of killing or greatly reducing the amount of bacteria, yeasts or molds on topical application.

---

2   These "free radicals" are toxic to certain molecules, cells, and tissues, which can lead to various disorders. The body often uses this toxicity to its own advantage, when immune cells are induced to generate free radicals to destroy bacteria or viruses.

Antistatic Agent: (See "Hair Conditioning Agent")

Aromatherapy: The art of using the pure essential oils of plants via baths, inhalation, massage or skin application, to create enjoyable and/or therapeutic experiences. The theory is that certain aromas alter brain waves and subconscious thought, and thereby affect learning, emotions, hormonal balances, release of chemicals from the brain and accelerate healing or emotional change.

Astringent: Ingredients that induce a tightening, firming, or tingling on the skin. Astringents, such as alum (potassium aluminum sulfate), cause a contraction of the skin and dry the skin. A product designated as a cosmetic astringent is likely to contain alcohol, aluminum compounds, natural tannins, or an herb such as witch hazel.

Barrier Agents: Wide variety of viscous and occlusive oily substances from vegetable, animal, mineral (silicones), or petroleum sources. They protect the skin from detergents, water, chemical irritants, and harsh climate. Used in creams and lotions and also in industrial preparations, typical barrier agents are occlusive ingredients such as petrolatum, silicones, and polymers. By themselves, they hold moisture in the skin very well, but tend to be aesthetically unpleasing (greasy or sticky). Therefore, they are usually used in creams and lotions at a lower percentage.

Beta Hydroxy Acids: A wide group of organic acids that function very similarly to alpha hydroxy acids. Studies show them to be very close in effectiveness when used for exfoliation. An example is salicylic acid.

Betaines: A group of cosmetic raw materials which generally exhibit properties similar to amphoterics. Betaines are employed as emulsifiers, cleansers, foaming agents, and skin and hair conditioners. Cocamidopropyl betaine, for example, is commonly used to make milder shampoos.

Biodegradable: Able to be decomposed by microorganisms. Specifically, the rate at which detergents, pesticides and other compounds may be broken down by bacteria and/or other environmental factors. The faster it breaks down into harmless products in the environment, the more biodegradable it is. There are a variety of regulations pertaining to what may or may not be termed "biodegradable." (The rules vary from country to country.)

Bioflavonoids: A phytonutrient group found in many fruits and vegetables with antioxidant and other medicinal properties. Necessary for proper capillary health.

Buffering Agent: An ingredient that can hold the pH of a liquid product within a narrow range even if small amounts of acids or bases are added. Used to maintain a product's pH at the desired level. (Also see: "pH Adjuster")

Carbohydrate: A compound of carbon, hydrogen, and oxygen in which the ratio of hydrogen to oxygen is the same as in water (2:1). Carbohydrates are the most abundant class of organic compounds, constituting three-fourths of the dry weight of all vegetation. They are also widely distributed in animals and in lower forms of life. They comprise (1) monosaccharides: simple sugars, such as fructose (levulose) and glucose (dextrose), both having the formula $C_6H_{12}O_6$; (2) disaccharides: sucrose ($C_{12}H_{22}O_{11}$), maltose, and lactose; and (3) polysaccharides (high polymeric substances). The last group includes the entire starch and cellulose families, as well as pectin, the seaweed products, agar and carrageenan, and natural gums. The simple sugars are crystalline and water-soluble, with a sweet taste; starches are water-soluble, tasteless and amorphous; cellulose is insoluble in water and organic solvents, and is only partially crystalline. Galactose, sorbose, zylose, arabinose, and manose are constituents of more complex sugars. The natural gums are water-soluble plant products composed of monosaccharide units joined by glycosidic bonds (arabic, tragacanth).

Carotenoids: A large group of phytonutrients (as many as 600), the best known of which is beta-carotene. Others are lycopene, alpha-carotene, lutein, and astaxanthin. They are the pigments that make up the colors in many fruits and vegetables. Particularly useful as antioxidants.

Cationic: Characterized by a positive charge on the hydrophillic (water soluble) portion of the molecule. Because this positive charge is attracted to negatively charged proteins in skin and hair, these materials are useful as conditioning agents. Quaternary ammonium compounds, as well as many hydrolyzed proteins, are a part of this group.

CFC: Chlorofluorocarbon. Used as aerosol propellants in cosmetic products until the late 1970s. Claimed to deplete the stratosphere of ozone.

CFR: Code of Federal Regulations. Contains the rules and regulations of the United States, including those applicable to personal care products and drugs.

Chelating Agents: Certain organic compounds are capable of binding metals (trace minerals which may contaminate a product). Such organic compounds are called chelating agents. The compound formed by a chelating agent and a metal is called a chelate. EDTA is a common chelating agent. Chlorophyll is a chelate that consists of a magnesium ion joined with a complex chelating agent. Heme, part of the hemoglobin in blood, is an iron chelate. Chelating agents soften water, prevent colors from fading, maintain the effectiveness of the preservative system, and prevent separation. (Also see: "Sequestering Agents")

Chemical: All matter is composed of chemicals. There is a tendency in the natural foods trade to use the term *chemical* as contrasted with another term: *natural*. The vagueness of the definition of both these words leaves the truly concerned consumer at a loss. We can no more turn away from chemicals that we could stop eating, drinking, breathing . . . these all require "chemicals." Our advice—ignore this word. It is often used to vilify certain ingredients or promote others. Focus on safety. (Also see: "Natural," "Organic," "Synthetic")

CIR: Cosmetic Ingredient Review. A panel evaluation of individual cosmetic ingredients, set up by the CTFA. Their findings are regularly published.

Cleanser: One of the primary functions of surfactants is cleansing. In order to do this, the cleanser must wet the body surfaces (see "Wetting Agent"), emulsify and solubilize oils, and suspend dirt. Cleansers also contribute foaming and lathering properties to cleansing products and bubble baths. Ingredients which are designated as cleansers include soaps, detergents and surfactants.

Soap is an alkaline cleanser. The surfactants, such as the lauryl or laureth sulfates, or betaines, are closer to the pH of skin.

Clinical Testing: Product testing done on human subjects, usually under controlled, clinical conditions.

Colloid: An extremely fine particle suspended in a surrounding medium. Not a solution, although frequently referred to as such, a colloid's particles are so fine that they will not normally settle out by gravity and they are small enough to be passed through most filters. Colloids may be a suspension of a solid in a gas (aerosol), a liquid in a liquid (emulsion), a solid in a liquid (suspension), a gas in a liquid (foam), or even a solid in solid. (Also see: "Emulsion")

Colorant: Color additives, coloring agents, and ingredients that impart color to the skin, hair or nails, or which are used to color finished products. Most colorants are synthetic in origin. Some (henna, annatto, some iron oxides and a few others) occur in nature. (Also see: "D&C Colors," "FD&C Colors," "Laked Colors")

The USFDA strictly regulates the pigments and dyes used in the U.S. cosmetic industry. The single biggest advantage of synthetic colors over natural colors is their superior stability. Natural colors are prone to fading or color change in many cases.

Comedogenic: Any ingredient or product that may be more likely to contribute to the formation of acne or blackheads (comedones). These may include irritants which provoke an internal response from the skin, occlusives which limit the skin's normal excretion and respiration, and oily or greasy ingredients which may attract and hold impurities to the skin's surface.

Conditioner: (See "Hair Conditioning Agents" or "Skin Conditioning Agents")

Cosmetic: As defined in the U.S. Federal Register, "Articles intended to be rubbed, poured, sprinkled or sprayed on, or introduced onto, or otherwise applied to the human body or any part thereof for cleansing, beautifying, promoting attractiveness, or altering the appearance, and articles intended for use as a component of any such articles; except that such term shall not include soap."

Note that soap was *excluded* from the regulations. That is why soap labels do not have to comply with the cosmetic labeling law.

Cream: From the cosmetic point of view, creams are essentially emollients. They are emulsions, usually of the oil in water (o/w) type. The heavier oily layer of the cream protects the skin by holding a film of water on the skin. It is the water and the substances in it which soften and moisturize the skin. The oily layer also protects the skin from the effects of the environment and can help keep the skin flexible in certain cases. Creams reduce flaking, lubricate, improve the appearance of the skin, and can help to mask the signs of aging. It is the active ingredients added to creams that produce specific additional effects. (Also see: "Humectant," "Occlusive," "Lotion")

CTFA: The Cosmetics, Toiletry and Fragrance Association, a private, industry organization. CTFA nomenclature found in the "CTFA *International Cosmetic Ingredient Dictionary*" (Sixth Edition, 1995), is the primary source for the names of cosmetic ingredients. The CTFA also establishes good manufacturing procedures for manufacturers of cosmetics and fragrances.

D & C Colors: Those colors approved by the U.S. FDA for use in drugs and cosmetics. Some contain coal tar dyes, whose safety is subject to evaluation. (Also see: "Colorant")

Each batch of D&C or FD&C color must be approved by the U.S. FDA before it can be sold to the cosmetic industry.

Deionized Water: (See "Water") This is the term given to water with most all of the hardness (calcium and magnesium) removed. Deionization is normally far from the final step in preparing water for product use.

In our own facility, and many others, the purification of water goes far beyond this, to include filtering, sterilization and impurity removal.

Demineralized Water: (See "Deionized Water")

Denaturant: Any number of substances which, when added to ethyl alcohol, makes it unfit for human consumption. Alcohol so treated usually has the letters "SD" (for Specially Denatured), before the word "alcohol."

Usually, that added substance is a "bittering" agent or something that makes it very unpalatable. (See appendix D.)

Deodorant: An ingredient or product that reduces or eliminates unpleasant odor on the body's surfaces. Deodorants work in a variety of ways. Absorbants can act as deodorants if they have the ability to absorb malodorous chemicals, and/or perfumes may be used to mask the odor. Chemical reactions can be used to neutralize the odoriferous substance in some cases, or a cosmetic biocide (such as lichen plant extract or tea tree oil) might be used to destroy or stop the formation of odor-causing microorganisms. Deodorants, unlike antiperspirants, do not interfere with the body's ability to perspire and as such, are not classified as drugs in the U.S.

Desquamation: The process by which the body sloughs off dead skin cells, that have keratinized and migrated to the skin's surface.

Detergent: A type of surfactant used in cleansing preparations. Any substance that reduces the surface tension of water, specifically, a surface-active agent which concentrates at oil-water interfaces, exerts emulsifying action, and thus aids in removing soil. The older and still widely used types are the common sodium soaps of fatty acids, which are relatively weak. The synthetic detergents are in four classes: amphoteric, anionic, cationic, or nonionic, depending on their mode of chemical action. The most widely used group comprises linear alkyl sulfonates (LAS), which are preferable to alkyl benzene sulfonates (ABS), because they are believed to be more readily decomposed by microorganisms (biodegradable). (Also see: "Surfactant")

Dispersion: A two-phase system in which one phase is a fine particle distributed throughout a surrounding second phase. The finer particle is the dispersed (internal) phase, the surrounding substance is the continuous (external) phase. A dispersion of a liquid in a liquid is an emulsion, a solid in a liquid is a suspension. Under normal conditions a dispersion is seldom uniform, but the addition of various surfactants such as wetting agents, dispersing agents, or emulsifiers will increase the uniformity.

Draize Test: A procedure to help evaluate the potential eye irritation of a product. Typically performed on rabbits.

Drug: As defined in the U.S. Federal Register, "Articles intended for use in the cure, mitigation, treatment, or prevention of disease in man . . . and articles (other than food) intended to affect the structure of any function of the body of man."

Emollient: A skin conditioning agent which helps maintain the smooth, soft, pliable appearance of skin. Emollients function by their ability to remain on the skin surface or in the stratum corneum (see "Skin") to act as lubricants, to reduce flaking, and to improve the skin's appearance.

Emulsifier: Most people know that oil and water don't mix—but there is a way. An emulsifier is a substance which enables oils or oil-soluble materials to be dispersed throughout a water base (or vice-versa) to form a cream or lotion. Emulsifiers are surfactants which speed or enable the formation of an emulsion. The emulsifier reduces the surface tension between the dispersed phase and the continuous phase, and they work in conjunction with emulsion stabilizers and thickeners (viscosity increasing agents). It usually requires more than one emulsifier to make an emulsion stable over the expected life of a product. (Also see: "Dispersion," "Emulsion")

Emulsion: Have you ever shaken up salad dressing with the oil on top and the water/vinegar on the bottom? Notice how they stay together, briefly? You created an emulsion for a brief moment. In cosmetics, an emulsion is a stable system in which two liquid systems which would normally not go into solution are held in suspension by a small percentage of one or more emulsifiers. The liquid in the dominant quantity is the continuous phase. the second liquid, held in uniform fine particles throughout the continuous phase, is called the dispersed phase. Creams and lotions are emulsions. (Without emulsification, the product would have two or three layers and require vigorous shaking before use.)

Emulsions are of two types, oil in water (o/w) and water in oil (w/o). Generally, heavier creams are w/o emulsions and lighter creams and lotions are o/w. Unlike colloids, emulsions may have a tendency to separate, requiring the use of emulsion stabilizers or thickeners (viscosity increasing agents) to support the function of the emulsifiers. (Also see: "Colloid," "Dispersion," "Micelle")

Eczema: Noncontagious skin condition characterized by redness, itchy scaling and sometimes, lesions. Frequently becomes encrusted.

Enzyme: Vital body catalysts that make possible or expedite certain critical chemical reactions in the body. For example, enzymes are required to digest food thoroughly. In skin care, they are sometimes used to help loosen and slough off dead skin cells in skin peels. They are now used in various medical treatments around the world.

Common examples are papain and bromelain.

Essential Oil: A volatile oil obtained from the leaves, stem, flower, or other parts of plants, usually carrying the odor characteristic of the plant. Most essential oils are mixtures, others are nearly pure single compounds (wintergreen oil is mostly methyl salicylate). Essential oils are not saponifiable, although they may be added to finished soaps or other products. Synthetic versions of many essential oils are available, largely due to the price and shortage of the supply of natural oils. The complexity and subtlety of each oil's mixture makes it very difficult, and in many cases, impossible to duplicate by synthetic means. In fact, essential oils of the same type plant, vary, depending on the source, type of extraction, crop conditions, time of the year it is harvested, climate and many other factors.

Ester: Organic compound formed by the reaction of an acid and an alcohol (or phenol). Usually liquid, usually fragrant. Esters of acetic acid are acetates, esters of carbonic acid are carbonates, esters of coconut fatty acids (lauric acid) are laurates. Esters can be solvents, surfactants, emulsifiers, emollients, conditioners and preservatives. Fatty esters (laurates, stearates, acetates, etc.) are commonly used in cosmetics and shampoos.

Ethoxylated: A process to reduce the irritation potential or improve the solubility of certain ingredients, surfactants in particular. For example, ammonium lauryl sulfate is more irritating than the related ethoxylate, ammonium laureth sulfate.

External (Ext.) D & C Colors: Colors certified by the U.S. FDA for external use only in drugs and cosmetics, not on lips or mucous membranes. (Also see: "D&C Colors," "FD&C Colors")

Exfoliant: A product or ingredient whose purpose is to remove dead skin cells, debris, or waste products from the skin and other body surfaces. Exfoliants are of three types: abrasives, enzymes or chemical peeling agents. (Also see: "Abrasives," "Enzymes")

Extract: A solution of plant oils or extracted plant material in water, alcohol, an alcohol-water mixture, or some other solvent such as glycerin or propylene glycol. Extracts can concentrate the oil or extracted material to several times the strength of the original plant material, but are not as concentrated as essential oils.

It is important to understand that the method of extraction is crucial in determining what is extracted from the herb. For example, water extraction yields only those components soluble in water, alcohol extraction removes only those materials soluble in alcohol, etc. Different extractions can yield very different extracts, containing very different ingredients.

Also be aware there are few standards. Legally, an extract can be whatever the supplier wants it to be. An investigation of the "actives" content is the only means of determining the components.

Fatty Acids: Natural components of vegetable and animal oils, fatty acids serve as the basic ingredient for soaps, surfactants, emulsifiers, foaming agents and many more cosmetic ingredients. Fatty acids are readily available from natural sources, including coconut, palm, safflower, soybean, sunflower, and other vegetable oils and animal fats. For this reason, synthetic fatty acids are not common.

Many emulsifiers and surfactants are produced from the fatty acids of coconut or palm oil. See the chart of oils and fats, and their fatty acid content in appendix B.

Fatty Alcohols: Prepared from fatty acids, fatty alcohols such as cetyl, stearyl or myristyl alcohol are used as emollients in numerous types of cosmetics. They also are co-emulsifiers, and are used to increase the viscosity of emulsions, shampoos and other products. Fatty alcohols are not drying and are *not* similar to grain alcohol (ethanol), which is a powerful solvent.

Fatty alcohols serve as the basis for the production of most shampoos and cleansing surfactants. For example, lauryl alcohol is used to make the lauryl sulfate cleansers. These fatty alcohols normally come from natural sources (coconut oil, for example), but can be synthesized in other ways.

FDA: The United States Food and Drug Administration, which became responsible for the regulation of the cosmetic industry under the Food, Drug and Cosmetic Act of 1938 and the enforcement of the Cosmetic Fair Packaging and Labeling Act. No cosmetic for consumer purchase produced after April 1977 may be filled into containers without full and accurate ingredient labeling, using standardized terms. (Also see: "CTFA")

Certain exemptions were made for "professional use only" product labels. For more information go to www.FDA.gov.

FD&C Colors: Certified by the FDA for use in food, drugs and cosmetics. Some are being reviewed for possible harmful effects. All FD&C Colors are synthetic, but not all are coal tar derivatives.

All batches produced must be approved by the FDA before shipment. (Also see: "Colorant")

Film Former: A material which is applied wet to the skin, hair or nails which produces a continuous film when dry. Used to form facial masks, make-up films, nail polish or hair holding products (such as hair spray polymers).

Flavonoids: A category of naturally occurring antioxidants, commonly found in fruits and vegetables. Sometimes referred to as "Vitamin P."

Formula: The list of ingredients and amounts or percentages that make up a personal care product (very similar to a recipe).

Fragrance: Any one of a wide range of essential oils or synthetic chemicals which impart a scent to the body or to the product. Some are intended to make the product more appealing, some are intended as perfume for the wearer. "Fragrance-free" products may contain no fragrance or may contain a small amount of a "masking" type fragrance. The consumer should check the product's ingredient list.

Fragrance may be listed by name or simply called "fragrance" in the list of ingredients. Nonetheless, it is usually a complex mixture of many volatile and reactive compounds, often more numerous than all the other ingredients in a cosmetic product. For this reason, if a person is sensitive to, or irritated by, a product, one likely cause is one or more of the fragrance ingredients.

Functional Ingredient: An ingredient designed for a specific function. It must be also understood that the functionality depends not only on the intrinsic activity of the molecule, but proper delivery of an adequate quantity of the ingredient to the site of action for a time period sufficient for it to perform well.

Gel: A semisolid liquid, often clear. Gels are common in shampoos, toothpastes and some skin care items.

Gum: A class of carbohydrates which swell in the presence of water and increase the thickness of water-based products. Gums are also used as suspending agents, gelling agents, and emulsion stabilizers. Some are useful in water-based lubricants.

Hair Colorant: Materials that impart color to the hair. These may be temporary, washing out easily, or semi-permanent, lasting through several shampooings, or permanent, unaffected by normal hair washing. How long any hair color lasts depends on the formulation and the skill of the stylist. Hair colorants are usually synthetic, although one natural material, henna, is the basis of many products.

Hair Conditioning Agent: Ingredients used to create an improved feel or special effects on hair. They repair or improve split ends, enhance manageability, improve "combability," appearance and feel of the hair, acting by adsorption as substantives. Others are antistatic electricity agents, preventing tangling or "fly-away" hair.

Humectant: A skin conditioning ingredient in creams and lotions whose function is to prevent water loss and drying of the skin. Humectants are hygroscopic, that is, they attract and hold moisture. In a moisturizer, they are intended to increase the water content of the top layer of the skin. Common examples are glycerin, propylene glycol, sorbitol, sodium PCA and the more expensive (and more effective) hyaluronic acid.

   Humectants also prevent or retard "shrinkage" of a cream itself by slowing water evaporation. Further, they can add to the ease of application of the cream.

   In extremely dry climates, some humectants can actually draw water from the skin. Proper formulation is essential for these climates.

Hydrocarbon: Compounds containing only hydrogen and carbon, usually derived from petroleum. Examples of plant derived hydrocarbons are azulene and squalane. Fruit and vegetable fatty acids contain hydrocarbon chains. Medium-weight liquids are widely used as emollients (mineral oil, petrolatum, squalene). Lower weight volatile hydrocarbon are solvents (mineral spirits, toluene), while gaseous hydrocarbons are used as propellants in aerosols (butane, propane). Many synthetic polymers are produced from hydrocarbons (polyethylene). Mineral oil and petrolatum are by far, the most frequently used petroleum hydrocarbons in cosmetics. There have been questions in the past about the purity and long term safety of petroleum hydrocarbons.

Hydrolysis: The process of breaking down larger molecules by means of acids, alkalies, heat and/or enzymes. For proteins, this means reducing the molecular weight, and the resulting smaller molecules are more water soluble.

Hydrolyzed Protein: Natural protein (animal, vegetable or milk) which has been broken down into more readily usable units and/or made soluble for use in cosmetics. Animal protein is similar in molecular structure to that of human hair.

   The protein is rendered water soluble by reacting the protein with an enzyme, acid or another method, which breaks the larger molecules into smaller molecules. These hydrolyzed proteins are effective as hair conditioners because of two qualities: adsorption and substantivity. In the dissolved state, hydrolyzed proteins can form a film over the hair and/or attach it to its surface (adsorption). The protein molecules exhibit a preference for the hair, and this attachment becomes relatively permanent (substantivity). Once attached to the hair, the hydrolyzed proteins are able to absorb moisture and help to moisturize the hair. It can protect the hair by forming a hard film over the cuticle, and can even help reinforce damaged hair, somewhat like a splint. In other words, the hair can appear thicker, more lustrous, and more manageable. (Also see: "Protein")

Hypoallergenic: A product which is less likely to cause adverse allergenic reactions than similar, competing products ("hypo" means "less," not "none"). This does not mean that the product will cause no reaction, just comparatively less reactions in the population overall. There is no legal definition at this time. It does *not* mean that someone who experiences an allergic reaction will have less of a reaction.

INCI: International Nomenclature Cosmetic Ingredient System. The current system of determining official names for cosmetic ingredients.

The following list[3] will help explain how molecular chain length relates to the naming system:

Carbons (main chain)	IUPAC[4] stem term	INCI fatty acids	INCI fatty alcohols
6	Hexane	Capric	Hexyl
7	Heptane	Heptanoic	Heptyl
8	Octane	Caprylic	Caprylyl
9	Nonane	Pelagronic	Nonyl
10	Decane	Capric	Decyl
11	Undecane	Undecanoic	Undecyl
12	Dodecane	Lauric	Lauryl
13	Tridecane	Tridecanoic	Tridecyl
14	Tetradecane	Myristic	Myristyl
15	Pentadecane	Pentadecanoic	Pentadecyl
16	Hexadecane	Palmitic	Cetyl
17	Heptadecane	Margaaric	Hepadecyl
18	Octadecane	Stearic	Stearyl
19	Nonadecane		
20	Eicosane	Arachidic	Arachidyl
21	Heneicosane		
22	Docosane	Behenic	Behenyl

---

3 From bibliography reference no. 6.
4 International Union of Physics and Chemistry.

Notes on Naming Ingredients:

Special Stems

Cosmetic ingredients often use raw materials that are a complex mixture of alkyl groups rather than a single fatty-chain material. When coconut oil is reacted to make a fatty alcohol, the resultant product is, in fact, a combination of various fatty alcohols. Instead of naming each alkyl group present, a stem term is used to reflect the source material. In this case, the fatty alcohols derived from coconut oil would be called coconut alcohol. Similarly, "soybean," "tallow" and "palm kernel" describe alcohols derived from these natural oils.

Derivatives

Derivatives, such as ethers and esters, can be named once the alkyl stem has been designated. An ether is composed of two hydrocarbon chains linked to an oxygen by single bonds. To name an ether, name each alkyl group and add "ether." Thus, an 18-C (stearyl) chain linked to a 16-C (cetyl) chain by an oxygen is stearyl cetyl ether.

Esters are the product of a carboxylic acid reacting with a fatty alcohol. They are named in three parts: the alkyl stem of the alcohol, the stem indicating the acid and the suffix "-ate." Thus, the ester formed by the reaction of cetyl alcohol and palmitic acid is cetyl palmitate.

Ingredient Statement: The list of ingredients on the outer container as required by regulations. Usually, size and placement is dictated by regulations, as in the United States.

Inorganic: In chemistry, the term inorganic refers to compounds which do not contain hydrocarbons and their derivatives. Inorganic can also refer to non-plant or non-animal source products, such as mineral type ingredients—clays, pumice, salts, etc. In cosmetics, the term organic and inorganic seldom refer to growing techniques as they do in the food industry. From the standpoint of natural personal care ingredients, there are many inorganic substances which are natural. Obvious necessities like air, water, carbon dioxide are inorganic chemicals. Prominent natural ingredients like iron oxides, sulfur and carbonates are all inorganic. Don't try to draw too much from this term as it applies to cosmetics, as it is used in many different ways. Assume that it means the ingredient is from non-plant, mineral sources and you will be correct most of the time.

Unless the manufacturer clearly states it as correct, do *not* assume that so-called organic products are organically grown, or that "inorganic" means it is not natural.

Intermediate: An organic compound that serves as a kind of "stepping stone" in a series of reactions which take the chemicals from initial ingredients to the final products.

Irritant: A substance that produces redness, itching, swelling or blisters on the skin. Unlike an allergen, an irritant has no systemic side effects and its effect is mostly related to the skin reaction.

In general, development of irritation depends on how intact or undamaged the skin (stratum corneum) barrier is. If it is intact and not dried or "defatted" (over-cleansed), it resists irritation much better. For example, products improperly formulated with too much sodium lauryl sulfate or improperly formulated cleansers can "de-fat" (remove protective oils) or impair the function of this barrier, making it more susceptible to irritation. Unique delivery systems such as liposomes, nanosomes, and special emulsions can reduce the irritation potential by minimizing skin exposure.

Further, there is some evidence that ethnicity can be an influence. There are reports that Asian skin is more sensitive to certain formulas than European skin. Light-complexioned persons of Celtic ancestry, who sunburn easily, also seem particularly vulnerable.

In cosmetics, the most common problem ingredient classes are certain preservatives and fragrances. (Natural fragrances are no exception.)

Other suspected ingredients are: water hardness (calcium), detergents and cleansers, solvents, some "quats," colors, and sunscreens. Items such as kola extract or caffeine are sometimes used as counter-irritants.

Keratin: A class of proteins that are not soluble (insoluble) in water and have characteristic hardness. Human nails, hair and skin are composed of keratin, as well as animal hooves and horns. Hydrolyzed keratin has been treated to make it water soluble by shortening the molecular chain length. (See "Hydrolyzed Protein")

Keratolyic Agent: Dissolves or loosens the intracellular material that causes cells to stick together, resulting in a sloughing off of the keratined dead skin cells on the top layers of the skin. This action can aid in combating acne and can also make the action of moisturizers more effective. Salicylic acid is a typical keratolyic agent.

Lake or (Laked) Colors: A pigment produced by precipitating an organic dye onto an underlying layer of an absorbent mineral. Insoluble in water, widely used as cosmetic make-up or lipstick colors. A wide range of colors, and numerous minerals are used as substrates—iron, calcium, copper, barium, and aluminum among them. The FD&C colors are usually used with an aluminum mineral substrate when changed into a "lake" color.

LD50 Testing: Used to determine the degree of toxicity of a product or raw material when ingested. LD50 is the lethal dose at which 50 percent of the organisms die.

Limonoids; Terpene substances, usually found in the peel of citrus fruits, which help protect against or fight disease in the body. (See "Terpenes")

Lipids/Lipoids: Fat and fat-like substances which occur in plants and animals. Lipids are a chief structural component of living cells. The term "lipid" is often used interchangeably with "fat" or "oil," and they are insoluble in water. (Also see: "Fatty Acid," "Oil")

Liposome: A double layer lipid which can be used to encapsulate a cosmetic ingredient. Liposomes are microscopic spheres resembling living cell membranes, which enables them to transport the ingredient deeper within the skin structure. Liposomes are sometimes claimed to promote the natural moisturizing function of the skin. In cosmetics, substances that could not normally be absorbed into the skin can sometimes be absorbed via liposomes. Different active ingredients will absorb at different rates.

It is not entirely understood how liposomes work, as they are at least as large as (or larger than), the skin's intracellular spaces. They may work by forming an occlusive layer on top of the released content of the liposome as it breaks on the skin surface.

Lotion: An emollient emulsion, usually of the oil in water (o/w) type. Lotions act as lubricants and help reduce flaking of dry skin. They are skin conditioning agents and often contain humectants and other active ingredients. Lotions and creams are similar in function, lotions being thinner (less viscous), less occlusive, with a smoother, less greasy feel on the skin. (Also see: "Cream," "Occlusive," "Humectant")

Mask: A cosmetic absorbent which, when mixed with water and allowed to dry on the skin, is intended to draw impurities from the skin's pores. Masks usually contain clay, kaolin, albumin or plant absorbents (starch, oat, rice) as their primary ingredients. To these, a variety of herbs, oils and other ingredients are frequently added to cleanse and soothe the skin.

MEA: (See "Alkanolamine")

Micelle: A kind of "super-emulsion" in which the emulsified, dispersed phase is surrounded by the maximum amount of emulsifier it can hold. This makes the micellized substance so small that it is more readily available on the skin for absorption by the body. Also sometimes referred to as "solubilization." This is a very superior form of emulsion and reduces the particles to the smallest size available, thereby increasing absorption. Micellized fat soluble nutrients and vitamins can be absorbed up to five times faster in the body.

Micelles are usually spherical in shape with the molecular polar group aligned towards the water phase and the non-polar group aligned towards the oil or non-polar phase. Liposomes are a form of micelle.

Microencapsulation: The surrounding of an ingredient by a film, shell or gelatin to protect that ingredient from the environment or to separate incompatible substances. The microcapsule breaks down by rubbing on the skin, or by way of the body's heat, oil, or moisture, This controls the release of ingredients or can help to extend the life of the product. (Also see: "Liposome")

Miscible: The ability of a gas or liquid to mix uniformly with another gas or liquid. All gases are completely miscible in other gases, but miscibility in liquids varies. Not all liquids are miscible in other liquids, i.e., water and oil are immiscible. Solids that mix completely with liquids are termed soluble rather than miscible, but the effect is the same.

Moisturizer: Any ingredient capable of moisturizing, combating dry skin or hair, or making the skin feel more moisturized. Some work by holding moisture in the skin (occlusive), others by providing water and water binding (hyaluronic acid), and some by providing oily substances to make the skin more flexible.

Literally, the term should mean adding water (moisture) to the skin. Marketing and advertising have taken us far past that definition.

MSDS: Material Safety Data Sheet. In the U.S., it is required to be in the premises of a manufacturer to alert workers to the potential dangers of individual raw materials.

Natural: Occurring in nature, whether of animal, vegetable or mineral origin. Usually does not refer to petroleum, its derivatives, or other chemically derived substances which are termed "synthetic." There is no accepted legal definition or standard for the word "natural" as it applies to a cosmetic product, so its presence on any label means only what the manufacturer intends it to mean. This meaning is frequently used to include "naturally derived," which is the processing of a substance which occurs in nature and/or its combination (reaction) with another ingredient. Most natural ingredients are filtered, purified, heated or processed in some fashion to achieve the desired end product. Sometimes the ingredient is reacted with another to achieve the desired effect, whether it be gentler, more effective, less irritating, etc.

The meaning is often interpreted as "safer than synthetic"—that may or may not be true. Personally, we prefer using natural ingredients that are time-tested safe, edible, and unlikely to cause a skin reaction. However, there are numerous instances when "natural" ingredients should be avoided in skin care. It is also safe to say there is no long history of time-tested safety for many of the synthetics and petroleum derivatives. Certain synthetic preservatives and fragrances are high on the list of likelihood to cause a skin reaction. (Also see: "Organic")

The only way this term can have real meaning for the consumer is to acquire the manufacturer's exact definition of his/her use of "natural," and compare it to his/her own.

NMF: An abbreviation for Natural Moisturizing Factor. NMF was first hypothesized in the 1930s, and described as a substance which exists in the human skin and keeps it supple. There is little evidence that NMF exists, nor is there a correlation between NMF and any single element in the skin. Furthermore, different manufacturers use the NMF description to mean different ingredients. NMF usually refers to a mixture of oils, humectants, and emollients similar to those found naturally in human skin oil (sebum).

Non-Alkaline: Having a neutral or acidic pH. (Also see: "Acid"; "pH")

Nonionic Surfactant: Characterized by a net neutral charge. Generally immune to the effects of pH, they provide flexibility in formulating. Can be good solubilizing agents.

Occlusive: A skin protecting agent which retards the evaporation of water from the skin's surface. By blocking the evaporative loss of water, occlusives increase the water content of the skin. Emollients are all somewhat occlusive to varying degrees. Occlusives will protect irritated or sensitive skin, and also protect skin against the effect of harsh environments (wind, cold, saltwater). They can, depending on which is used and how much is used, also inhibit the skin's natural respiration, clog pores, and be comedogenic. The most common occlusives are petrolatum, mineral oil and some polymers. Intelligent formulation requires careful selection of occlusives.

Oil: A generic name applied to a wide range of substances, many of which are quite different. Oils derived from plants or animals are usually mixtures of fatty acids such as oleic, palmitic, stearic, lauric, etc. They are used as primary ingredients in cosmetics as lubricants and emollients, and they are frequently saponified to yield glycerin and fatty acid soaps. The fatty acid soaps produced by saponification are themselves the raw materials for some cosmetic ingredients. The only difference between oils and fats is that oils generally have a shorter chain length molecule, and stay liquid at room temperature.

Hydrocarbon oils, such as mineral oil, petrolatum, jojoba and squalane are quite different in structure than fatty acid fruit and vegetable oils. Essential oils are very different, complex mixtures of organic oils.

Oil Phase: The oil soluble or non-polar components of an emulsion.

Organic: From a chemistry viewpoint, organic refers to all compounds containing carbon with a few simple exceptions (carbon oxides, carbonates, carbon sulfides and a few metallic carbon compounds). Carbon is present in every cell of every plant which is living or has been alive. This includes all petroleum substances which, although now inert, were derived from once-living organisms.

The term organic is entirely different when applied to agriculture. You must find out from the manufacturer what he/she means by the use of the word "organic." In cosmetics almost all ingredients are "organic," even though some may be synthetic (derived from petrolatum).

This term is often used to make an ingredient or formula appear to be what it is not. Ask the manufacturer for his clear definition of this word. It may likely not mean "organic" as used in the food industry. (Also see "Inorganic")

OTC (Over the Counter) Drugs: There are about ten categories of ingredients for externally used cosmetic products for which drug claims can be made and which can be sold without a prescription. An OTC drug uses a different format for listing ingredients, with the drug ingredient(s) listed as "Active Ingredients" at the beginning. If you are using sunscreens, fluoride toothpaste, or antiperspirants, then you are using OTC drugs. It is important to note that an ingredient can have a dual use— sometimes as a drug, sometimes as a non-active ingredient, e.g. salicylic acid is a drug when used as an acne medication, it is not if it is used as an exfoliant. Sunscreens containing PABA or benzophenones are OTC drugs, but these same ingredients can be used as UV absorbers in a non-drug application.

If you wonder how a cosmetic ingredient can also be a "drug" ingredient, you are not alone. Many believe the FDA regulations, based on advertising claims, are archaic.

Pearlizing Agent: Contributes an opaque, glossy or shiny "pearl" appearance to a product.

PEG: (POE, Polyoxyethylene, polyethylene glycol, ethoxylated, etc.) This is a prefix used or a suffix added, to indicate that a particular molecule has been modified by the attachment of a polymer chain of ethylene oxide. This is normally done to improve solubility characteristics, mildness or emulsifying properties. Generally, the larger the number, the longer the chain, and the more water soluble it is. The number associated with it indicates the amount of polymer added (PEG-10, for example).

Many manufacturing techniques can be utilized to make these attachments. Some older methods left free ethylene oxide and/or 1,4-dioxane (a suspected carcinogen) in the ingredient. Currently, there are procedures available that eliminate these potentially dangerous by-products and are they are normally now utilized for most ingredients intended for food, drug, or cosmetic use. Again, it is up to the manufacturer of the product to insure that PEGs are properly prepared and free of contaminants.

Petroleum: Crude oil as pumped from the earth. Although "natural" and "organic," it may contain substances best not used on the skin. Mineral oil, petroleum and tar are all "fractions" (parts) of this complex mixture.

pH: A scale from 0 to 14 used in measuring acidity or alkalinity of solutions. pH 7.0 is considered neutral. Acidity increases as the numbers decrease below 7.0, while alkalinity increases as the numbers increase above 7.0. The normal pH of skin and hair is between 4.0 and 6.0, slightly acidic. The pH of a product is important for many reasons. Some examples: If the pH of a shampoo is too alkaline, the hair may be damaged; if it is too acidic, the shampoo will not cleanse properly. Many ingredients function best in a certain pH range. For example, for certain preservative systems to work properly, the pH must be held within a narrow range. (Also see: "pH Adjuster")

pH Adjuster: An ingredient used to control the pH of a finished cosmetic product. pH adjusters alter the product's pH and maintain it at the desired level. (Also see: "Buffering Agent")

Common pH adjusters include citric acid, lactic acid, triethanolamine, potassium hydroxide and sodium hydroxide. (Usually used at well below 1 percent of the total product weight.)

Photosensitization: The process by which a substance or organism becomes sensitive to light. Some cosmetic ingredients can be photosensitizers.

In dermatology, the process that causes an allergic response in an individual when a chemical is exposed to light. Certain essential oils can result in a photosentization reaction in sunlight.

Phytonutrients: Essential nutrients—vitamins, minerals, antioxidants and others—derived from plants.

Polymer: Natural or synthetic macromolecules formed by the repetition of an identical, smaller molecule or group of molecules. Silicone is an inorganic, natural polymer. Cellulose and gums are plant-based polymers, and keratin and DNA are protein polymers. Synthetic polymers in cosmetic chemistry are numerous and diverse (i.e. carbomer, PEG).

Polysaccharide: Found in nature as the structural and protective materials in plants and animals, or the reserve nutrients. Examples are cellulose, starch, alginates, hyaluronic acid (a mucopolysaccharide), gum arabic, carrageenan (from algae and seaweed), and chitin from crustacean shells.

In animals, they are found in joint fluids and cartilage.

PPG: (POP, propoxylated, polypropylene glycol) This is a prefix used to identify a material modified by the attachment of a polymer chain of propylene oxide, to improve solubility characteristics or emulsifying properties. The number associated with it indicates the amount of polymer added. (PPG-10, for example)

Preservative: Cosmetics are subject to contamination and deterioration in many ways. A preservative system, in order to be completely effective, must be able to prevent the growth of bacteria, yeast, mold, and fungus. The preservative system must also prevent oxidation (rancidity), and in some cases it must retard separation and discoloration of the product. Most preservatives are effective in very small concentrations (0.01–0.8 percent of the volume of the product). Two or more preservatives working together as a system can actually reduce the total amount of preservative needed. This occurs because they each may be more effective in specific activity, and because they heighten each other's efficacy due to synergistic effects.

Knowledgeable chemists often use lesser amounts of two or three preservatives, as opposed to a larger amount of a single preservative. This can make the system more effective *and* lessen the chance for irritation.

In very high concentrations (usually exceeding approximately 15–20 percent), alcohol, propylene glycol, glycerin and honey have preservative functions. Even then, they may not be completely effective. Very low pHs can also assist in preventing growth of microorganisms.

Protein: A complex polymer containing carbon, hydrogen, oxygen, nitrogen, and usually sulfur, and comprised of chains of amino acids. Proteins occur in the cells of all living organisms and in biological fluids (blood, plasma, protoplasm). They are synthesized by plants largely because of the nitrogen-fixing ability of certain soil bacteria. Their molecular weight may be as high as 40 million (tobacco mosaic virus). They have many important functional forms: enzymes, hemoglobin, hormones, viruses, genes, antibodies, and nucleic acids. They also comprise the basic component of connective tissue (collagen), hair (keratin), nails, feathers, skin, etc. Some have been synthesized in the laboratory.

Proteins can be broken down into polypeptides and these, in turn, can be hydrolyzed down to their constituent amino acids. They form colloidal solutions, and behave chemically as both acids and bases simultaneously (See "Amphoteric"). They can be denatured by changes in pH, by heat, ultraviolet radiation and many organic solvents.

Although contained in skin and hair, there is little proof that protein in shampoos or creams actually alters the structure of the hair or skin. Proteins work by coating the skin or hair, and by attaching themselves (via cationic charge) to the hair and making it feel smoother, easier to comb and adding "body." On the skin, they attract moisture and make the skin feel smoother.

Pure: This word can mean almost anything a manufacturer wishes it to mean. It could be applied to single (full strength) ingredient products (such as 100 percent tea tree oil), it could mean that certain contaminants have been removed from the ingredients or formula, or it could imply that certain contaminants are not present in the formula. Don't put too much faith into this word. Ask the manufacturer what they mean by its use if you are curious.

Focus on safety and effectiveness.

Psoriasis: Common, chronic, recurrent skin disease characterized by patches of flaking and/or discolored skin, believed to affect 1–3 percent of the American population.

Purified Water: Water purified to meet the requirement of certain U.S. Drug Regulations. It is not a proper cosmetic ingredient listing. (Also see: "Water")

Quaternary Ammonium Compounds: (AKA: "Quats") A large group of cationic surfactants comprised of a central nitrogen atom surrounded by four organic groups and an acid radical. Wide variety of uses, depending upon the compound, including disinfectant, hair conditioner, cleanser, sterilizer, preservative, deodorant, and wetting agent. Quats are useful because the nitrogen is positively charged, causing it to be attracted to the protein in skin and hair. They are often used as conditioners in this manner. Quaternization increases the substantivity of an ingredient, enabling it to remain on the skin or hair when other water soluble ingredients might be rinsed away. Benzalkonium chloride, cetrimonium bromide and chloride, stearalkonium chloride, and polyquaterniums are all examples of quats.

Raw Materials: The ingredients used to make personal care products, no matter what type or source.

Rinse: Usually refers to a class of hair conditioning agents which are primarily antistatic agents, providing good detangling, ease of combing and preventing "fly-away" hair. Usually, the active ingredients used are "quats." (See "Quaternary Ammonium Compounds")

Rubefacient: A substance that causes a reddening of the skin by increasing the blood supply to it (Example: pepper oil [capsaicin], niacin, niacinamide, cinnamon oil, etc.)

Salt: The chemical combination of an acid and a base yields a salt plus water. Table salt is sodium chloride (NaCl), and is formed by the following reaction: HCl (hydrochloric acid) + NaOH (sodium hydroxide) = NaCl + H2O.

Soap is a type of salt which is formed by the reaction between a fatty acids and a metallic alkali (base). Remember that "salt" is a very broad term in chemistry, encompassing many types of ingredients, and organic salts can be very diverse and complex. (See "Saponification")

Saponification: The combination of an alkali, usually sodium hydroxide (lye) or potassium hydroxide (caustic potash), and a fatty acid. The salt formed is called a soap. Most of the caustic nature of the alkali disappears because two entirely new compounds are formed in an irreversible reaction. In the case of lye, all the sodium is contained within the soap, the hydroxide in glycerin, the major by-product of saponification. Soaps formed in this manner are alkaline, and not recommended for good skin and hair care. (Also see: "Soap")

Saponins: Widely occurring in natural glycosides, which will form a soapy lather when combined with water and agitated. Found in many plants, including saponaria, sarsaparilla, soapbark, wild pansy, etc. They foam, emulsify, and reduce surface tension. Used in soaps, shampoos, shaving creams. Generally not toxic to skin, some saponins are anti-irritants.

Yucca juice, for example, contains natural saponins and can be used as a foaming/cleansing agent.

Saponins are not normally used as prime surfactants due to their weak cleansing ability, high price and poor supply problems.

The saponins in soybeans may have cholesterol-lowering effects and some anti-cancer properties.

Sarcosinates, Sarcosine Derivatives: A class of derivatives of fatty acids. They form anionic surfactants primarily used for skin or hair cleansing applications. Useful at lower pH (less alkaline) than more alkaline cleansers, they are generally less drying, less irritating and more substantive.

Sensitizer: A substance which initially acts as an antigen, producing an immune response within the body. It is only later—whether a second exposure or after a series of exposures extending over years—that the body has a powerful secondary response. This is an intense and usually sudden allergic response, far greater than ordinary allergies.

Photoallergic dermatitis is a type of sensitization.

Examples of potential sensitizers are: some fragrances, certain preservatives, some hair dyes (p-phenylenediamine), lanolin, glyceryl thioglycolate, toluenesulfonamide/formaldehyde resin (in some nail polishes) and some sunscreens.

Sequestering Agents: Certain organic compounds are capable of reacting with various metals to prevent physical and chemical changes within the final product; such organic compounds are called sequestering agents. Sequestering agents bind up metallic ions, making water "softer." In a shampoo this prevents dull films and the hair appears shinier. They can also protect a product by preventing physical changes affecting color, flavor, texture, or appearance. Sequestering agents act along with antioxidants to help preserve the original product characteristics. (Also see: "Chelating Agents")

Shampoo: As a cleansing preparation for hair, a shampoo is basically a water solution of a surfactant with good cleansing and foaming properties. In this function, the surfactant or combination of surfactants should wet the hair and scalp (see wetting agents), emulsify or solubilize oils, and suspend soil. There is no need for the shampoo to foam or lather, but users find these properties reassuring, and foam-boosters are a common part of modern shampoo formulations. Commercial shampoos were unknown before the 1930s, and the earliest products were either liquid soap-based, or used some of the harsher synthetic surfactants. Modern shampoos are a mixture of gentle acidic surfactants, as soaps leave a dulling film on the hair. Blends of herbs are also frequently added for their traditional benefits. Fragrance, color, thickeners, and preservatives are also common. (Also see: chapter 3, pages 27–29)

Silicones: Polymers made from silica (silicon dioxide or sand), they are used to help the product "spread" easily, and to protect the skin.

Skin: The external covering of the human body, including the hair growing through it. Skin has two general layers. The epidermis is the outer layer. Its surface is the stratum corneum, comprised of the hard, keratinized dead cells which are held together by a mortar-like mixture of water, fatty acids, ceramides, cholesterol and squalane and other lipids. The stratum basale, at the base of the epidermis, is a germative layer: each day a new layer is formed and each day a dead layer is sloughed off the surface of the stratum corneum. Although the epidermis has no blood vessels or nerves, it does contain enzymes and hormones, and it is considered a living tissue due to its continual differentiation.

The dermis is the skin's second layer. It is below the basal layer of the epidermis, provides nutriment to the epidermis, cushions the body against mechanical damage, and it is the larger portion of the skin. Glands, hair follicles, blood and lymphatic vessels, and nerves are all located in the dermis, which is largely comprised of connective tissue: collagen, elastin, and mucopolysaccharides. Beneath the dermis is a layer of subcutaneous fat. (See pages viii, 38.)

Moisturizing the skin is best achieved when the stratum corneum is softened and saturated. It is now well accepted that many chemicals are able to enter the body by penetration through the skin. (Also see: "Moisturizer," "Humectant," "Emollient," "Skin Conditioning Agent," "Skin Protectant")

The skin is the body's largest organ, with a total area of about 18,000 square centimeters and weighs approximately 4.8 kilograms (about 10 pounds) in the average adult.

Skin Conditioning Agent: Designed to improve the feel or appearance of the skin. Emollients, humectants, occlusives, proteins, quats, or substantives are all skin conditioning agents. (See all)

Skin Protectant: Officially, an active ingredient in an OTC drug that is defined by the FDA as "a drug which protects injured or exposed skin or mucous membrane surface without harmful or annoying stimuli."

Unofficially, the term applies to any ingredient used to protect, prevent serious moisture loss, treat burns or rashes, etc.

Soap: A compound formed by combining a fat or an oil with a caustic alkali (see "Saponification"). The fatty component may be tallow, lard, olive oil, coconut oil (or any of its constituent oils), or a host of other fatty acid oils. The alkali is usually sodium hydroxide (lye) in the manufacture of bar or solid soaps, or potassium hydroxide or triethanolamine, in the manufacture of liquid soap. The production of extra creamy or super-fatted soaps is achieved by adding extra oils back in as the soap is cooling. A wide range of colors, fragrances, deodorizing or other medicinal ingredients, antibacterials, or other additives are added to the basic soap, in the final stages of manufacture. Soaps are alkaline (high pH), and do not lather well in hard water. They are wetting agents which form bonds with dirt, effectively removing and suspending dirt and oil from skin or fabrics. Some soaps can be irritating on sensitive skin. Fatty acid produced soap is not regarded as a cosmetic by the FDA, and is therefore not required to list ingredients on its package.

Solubilizer: A type of surfactant used to completely disperse (and solubilize) an insoluble ingredient. Solubilizers are commonly used to help fragrance oils into solution, to produce clear products.

Solution: A mixture of mutually soluble components. Table salt in water, for example, will form a completely clear solution until it reaches the maximum solubility of the salt at a particular temperature.

Solvent: Liquids or solids used to dissolve other ingredients. Water is the most common, and is called the universal solvent. Alcohols with a low molecular weight (ethyl, isopropyl, etc.), oils, glycerin and propylene glycol, are also frequently-used solvents. A solvent may be necessary in formulating a product, or it may be the function of the product, such as removing sebum from the skin, removing make-up, etc.

SPF: Sun Protection Factor. A rating of a product's effectiveness as a sunscreen. It is not an absolute rating which tells a user how much time is safe in the sun. Rather, the rating is relative to the user's own sensitivity to ultra-violet light. An SPF of two doubles the time an individual could be safe from burning under certain conditions, a SPF of ten means that they are safe for ten times as long, etc. Originally the scale of SPF only extended as high as 15, but manufacturers have chosen to describe some products with far higher numbers.

For example, if one could normally stay in the sun for 15 minutes, unprotected, without burning, the use of an SPF-10 should allow 15 minutes X 10, or 150 minutes without burning. In reality, due to perspiration, activities, skin rubbing against clothing, etc., it is always best to reapply a sunscreen frequently.

Caution: Sun is one of the greatest causes of premature aging and skin cancer. Do not allow the "feeling of invincibility" that often comes from sunscreen use to lull you into believing long term damage cannot take place. You can have serious effects without getting a sunburn. There is evidence that the more sun to which you are exposed during your lifetime, the more likely you are to suffer premature aging. The effect is cumulative.

Static Flyaway: Hair in a state of disarray due to a build-up of static electricity on the hair, causing individual hair shafts to repel each other. More common in dry, low humidity climates.

Stearates: A group of fatty acid derivatives (the esters, or soaps, of stearic acid), used to help produce emulsions in creams and lotions. They can be of vegetable, animal or synthetic origin.

Sterols: Solid alcohols from animals or plants. Cholesterol (or cholesterin) is a sterol used as a lubricant in creams or lotions. Soya sterols from soybeans, for example, are excellent emulsifiers and moisturizers for the skin.

Stratum Corneum: The outermost barrier layer of skin, primarily composed of dead, keratinized cells with no nucleus. This top layer of cells is completely cut off from the body's circulation and is unable to absorb nutrients. It is, however, not inert, and it is important for proper skin functioning and hydration. Also believed to modulate many enzymic activities that go on in the upper layers of the skin. Many surfactants and even prolonged exposure to plain water can disrupt its barrier function. One goal of cosmetics is to keep the stratum corneum moisturized (hydrated) so that it functions properly and feels smooth.

Substantive: An ingredient which, when it is applied to the skin or the hair, is adsorbed onto the skin or hair and is not easily removed, or does not easily rinse off. The substantive exhibits a preference for the surface onto which it is adsorbed, and acts to protect and strengthen the hair or skin, or give it an improved feeling on the surface.

For example, hydrolyzed proteins and quats are substantive to hair and not easily removed. Some sunscreen lotions are substantive to skin because they form a film that resists being removed with water.

Substantivity: The degree or property of being substantive.

Sulfated Fatty Acids and Alcohols: Originally introduced in the 1930s, these resulted in the first widespread popularity of soapless shampoos. Sodium Lauryl Sulfate had always been the most commonly used, because it is the most soluble, an excellent cleanser, and produces the most lather. In the last few years, its milder ethoxylate, sodium laureth sulfate, has become more widely used.

Sunscreen: The active ingredient in an OTC drug or cosmetic which protects the user from the effects of ultra-violet (UV) light. These effects include the burning in the UVB range, and aging and skin cancer in the UVA range. A sunscreen's effectiveness against UVB is rated by SPF, but there is no rating for effectiveness against UVA. PABA (para-aminobenzoic acid) and octyl dimethyl PABA were, until recently, the most widely used sunscreens. Newer, less likely to irritate, sunscreens are octyl methoxycinnamate, benzophenone and titanium dioxide. (See "SPF")

The FDA definition of a sunscreen is, "an active ingredient (from the approved list) that absorbs, reflects or scatters radiation in the UV range at wavelengths from 290 to 400 nanometers." Sunscreens are effective because they convert the UV light into infra-red radiation (heat) and reflect light. Standards for water-resistant and waterproof (very water resistant) sunscreens are also established. The former must remain effective for at least 40 minutes when exposed to water, the latter must remain effective for eighty minutes. More detail is available from the FDA website (www.FDA.gov).

Sunscreens function best when they remain *on* the skin surface, as opposed to being absorbed. As of this writing, the USFDA has approved only 16 ingredients for use as a sunscreen. In the U.S., it is not permitted to use any others until they are officially approved and added to the list. Therefore, all sunscreen formulas will contain sunscreens from this list. (Also see: chapter 3, pages 34, 35, and 40)

Surface Active Agent: (See "Surfactant")

Surfactant: A compound that reduces the surface tension in water, between water and another liquid, or between liquid and a solid. Surfactants form a large group of cosmetic ingredients, with a variety of important functions. They are commonly divided by function into cleansing agents, emulsifying agents, foam boosters, hydrotropes, solubilizing agents, and suspending agents. Surfactants, which are all wetting agents to varying degrees, are classified on the basis of their ionizing characteristics. Cationics (positive charge) are used as antistatic friction reducers in hair rinses and texturizers in skin creams. Anionics (negative charge) are strong cleansing agents. Nonionics (neutral ionic charge) are good grease cutters and solubilizers. Amphoterics are able to have either a positive or a negative charge (able to function either as an acid or a base), depending on the nature of the product. They are used in the most gentle cleansers, shampoos, and lotions. Many surfactants are derived from coconut oil or palm kernel oil, but there are many synthetic surfactants as well. New sources include surfactants derived from a variety of plant oils, including babassu, rice bran, avocado, cocoa butter and wheat germ.

This is a general term applied to a very large number of non-soap cleansers and emulsifiers. In and of itself, it does not imply mildness or lack thereof.

Synthetic: An ingredient or other chemical which either duplicates a natural substance, or which is a unique material not found in nature. Most synthetic ingredients are organic (in the chemistry sense of the word) and derived from petroleum.

TEA: (See "Alkanolamine")

Terpenes: Complex hydrocarbons. Most volatile or essential oils contain terpenes, many as the active ingredients in those essential oils. Some of the more common terpenes used in cosmetics are carotenes, limonoids and saponins. Commonly found in fruits and vegetables, they have a wide variety of functions in the body—antioxidants, protectors, hormone modifiers, blockers of cholesterol absorption, eye protectors and many other effects beneficial to cells.

Thickening Agent: (See "Viscosity Increasing Agent")

Toxic: A danger to the body. Everything, including oxygen and water, at some level becomes toxic. This word is often misused or misunderstood. For our purposes, we will use it to describe ingredients only at the levels commonly found in skin and hair care products. Arsenic, for example, has been used in certain cancer treatments. We would rate it toxic at anything but an extreme trace level in skin care. Selenium is a vital trace mineral, but it too, is toxic at higher levels. Concentration is the key fact in determining toxicity. (See pages 17–20)

Unscented: The term does not necessarily mean there is no fragrance present. This could mean: (1) There is no fragrance at all in the product; (2) There is no added fragrance in the product (it has a naturally occurring odor due to its ingredients); (3) There is no artificial fragrance added; natural essential oils are used; or (4) A very small amount of a "masking"-type fragrance was used.

You can usually tell from the ingredient list. If not, ask the manufacturer. (Also see: "Fragrance")

UV Absorber: Ultraviolet (UV) light is not only damaging to your skin, it can also cause physical or chemical deterioration of cosmetic products. UV absorbers are ingredients which protect the product from the loss of stability, deterioration and color fading caused by UV light. Sunscreens and UV absorbers are frequently the same, but when the ingredient is used as a sunscreen, the product is usually an OTC drug. Like sunscreens, UV absorbers have the ability to convert UV radiation into infrared radiation (heat).

Viscosity Increasing Agent: An ingredient used to thicken cosmetic products. Some are effective in water solutions like shampoos or other emulsions; salt (sodium chloride), alginates, gum tragacanth, gum karaya, carbomer, clays, polymers or cellulose gums are examples. Others are used to thicken the lipid (oily) portion of a product, like lipstick or pastes (cetyl alcohol or waxes are used, for example). Viscosity increasing agents are important for keeping the product thick enough to use as intended, and also for maintaining the thickness needed for the package type to be effective.

VOC: Volatile organic compound. Recent regulation at the state level has restricted the use of those ingredients, for the purpose of complying with the U.S. EPA clean air standards. Examples are hydrocarbon aerosol propellants and ethanol in hair sprays and deodorants.

Federal regulations are currently being developed.

Water: The inorganic compound of hydrogen and oxygen, H_2O. The most common cosmetic ingredient, and the most widely used solvent. In order for a product to be consistent and made to standards, the water itself must be standardized. This requires sterilized water, because microorganisms in the formula might multiply rapidly and spoil the product; purified and/or filtered water, because suspended contaminants must be removed; de-mineralized water because minerals in water (hard water) impede or cause chemical reactions. Since the normal pH of water is about 7.0, excess alkalinity or acidity must be neutralized or the product's stability cannot be assured. If the water is not properly purified, the final product may vary from batch to batch, may become contaminated, may discolor, or may separate.

Water is the first ingredient in most shampoos, rinses, conditioners, lotions, and other liquid products. The ingredient should read "water" but euphemisms abound: spring water, rainwater, barley water, purified water, herbal water, etc. While it is understandable that the manufacturer wants to make the product sound more natural and more desirable, the consumer should know that water is water . . . no more, no less. Technically, if a product ingredient list includes something like "herbal extract of . . ." that ingredient list should also list the solvent used to extract it. In many cases, it may be water, and it may be that the herbal content of this ingredient is not as important as the fact that it is the source of water for the finished product.

As innocuous as water seems, it too can be an irritant. There is speculation this occurs because of pH, occlusive properties, changes in the skin's micro environment, permitting of penetration of foreign substances and/or other factors.[5]

---

5   See bibliography, reference 9 for more information.

Water Phase: The part of an emulsion containing the water and water-soluble ingredients.

Wax: A low melting organic mixture or compound of high molecular weight, normally solid at room temperature and generally similar in composition to fats and oils except that it contains no glycerides. Some are hydrocarbons; others are esters of fatty acids and alcohols. They are usually classified among the lipids. Waxes are thermoplastic, but since they are not high polymers, they are not considered in the family of plastics. Common properties are water repellency, smooth texture, non-toxicity, freedom from objectionable odor and color. They are often combustible, and have good dielectric properties. Soluble in most organic solvents; insoluble in water. The major types are as follows:

I.   Natural
    1.   Animal (beeswax, lanolin, shellac wax, Chinese insect wax)
    2.   Vegetable (carnauba, candelilla, bayberry, jojoba, rice bran wax)
    3.   Mineral
        a.   Fossil or earth (ozokerite, ceresin, montan)
        b.   Petroleum waxes (paraffin, microcrystalline)
II.   Synthetic
    1.   Ethylenic polymers and polyl ether-esters ("Carbo-wax")
    2.   Chlorinated napthalenes ("Halowax")
    3.   Hydrocarbon type via Fischer-Tropsch process (synthetic jojoba oil, synthetic beeswax, synthetic wax)

Uses: Various waxes are found in all types of cosmetics to impart high viscosity to emulsions and suspensions and to harden lipid-based materials, such as lipsticks and hairdressings.

Wetting Agent: A surfactant. In a solution, it reduces the surface tension of water. This allows the water to penetrate into or onto another material, or to spread more completely over its surface. In a sense, a wetting agent makes the water "wetter." Soaps, fatty alcohols, and fatty acids and all surfactants are wetting agents, but the definition is generally reserved for wetting agents which are used specifically and uniquely for that purpose. (Also see: "Surfactants")

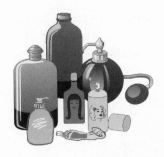

Chapter 7

Ingredient Dictionary

First, a word of explanation of names, symbols and rating numbers.

1. Ingredient Names

INCI[1]—official name as required on the label (most are the same as their CTFA[2] name).

Other names—common or trade names, not permitted on the label, but often used in other sources of information. (These names or terms are in parentheses or will refer you to the INCI name.)

2. Source Codes

Source codes tell you from where the product is derived. In many cases, there is more than one source. In those instances, we have listed the most common source where there is clearly a most common usage. In cases where more than one source is commonly used, we have listed all the sources.

A Animal
V Vegetable
M Mineral
S Synthesized
P Petrochemical Source (from Crude Oil)
H Human Source

---

1   International Nomenclature of Cosmetic Ingredients
2   Cosmetic, Toiletry and Fragrance Association

Many ingredients will have more than one source. On labels where you see these ingredients, only the manufacturer can advise you of the ingredient source. (This is another reason why I recommend using only one or two manufacturers, from whom you have already received assurances in this area, if it is important to you.) We have used our opinion where natural source ingredients have been processed or reacted to form a second ingredient. We understand that purists and others may disagree in some cases, as it is difficult to define exactly when a natural ingredient stops becoming "natural" in the process.

Please send us your recommended changes along with an explanation, for inclusion in future editions.

3. Purpose Codes

E Emulsifier

Exf Exfoliant (Removes dead skin cells via abrasion or chemical action)

M Moisturizer or Emollient

P Preservative or Antibacterial

T Thickener

F Fragrance or Flavor

C Color

CL Cleanser/Cleansing surfactant

S Stabilizer (To make the emulsion more stable and/or produce a longer shelf life)

A Active Ingredient— Special Use

Sol Solvent (To dissolve another ingredient or act as the base for the entire product. For example: water, alcohol, etc.)

O Antioxidant

pH Used to adjust the pH (acidity/alkalinity) of a product

AB Abrasive

4. *Safety Ratings*

In this section you will get my opinion (in concert with that of my consulting chemists) based on the data we found, testing results, official compendia, CTFA information, available technical articles and a great many years of personal experience. We respect the fact that there may be conflicting opinions for some materials. Please feel free to send us your suggestions for changes in future editions.

Rather than confuse consumers with the information for the pure raw material as is often done, we have confined our ratings to the percentage commonly found in personal care products. We recognize there may be extreme products in the marketplace. For example, our comments about AHAs cannot possibly cover every concentration one might find in the marketplace, especially one at an extremely high levels.

Another issue to consider is, what about an ingredient that tends to cause skin irritation at lotion concentrations above 5 percent, almost no reaction below that level, and none in a rinse-off product? I have tried to take care of this in the "notes" section. Always remember that the *concentration* (percentage) is crucial to the determination of irritation potential. Also, be aware the certain ingredients can be made less irritating (or more) by the addition of other ingredients. "Leave-on" products like moisturizers are more likely to irritate than "rinse-off" products such as shampoos.

There is no substitute for informed, intelligent formulation. Further, information about a particular raw material ingredient may have no bearing on the safety of the final formula.

In the end, we tried to take the most conservative position when ambiguities or differences occurred in opinion and literature. The guiding approach was—*what would we recommend to our own family?*

Abbreviations Used

>   greater than
<   less than
RO "Rinse off" products (bath gels, shampoos, etc.)
LV "Leave on" products (moisturizers, sunscreens, etc.)

Overall Safety Ratings (*S*) of Ingredients

1—Extremely safe—probably edible
2—Very safe as normally used in cosmetics
3—Safe as normally used in cosmetics
4—Some reported problems—may depend on the level
5—Avoid

Likelihood of an Ingredient to Cause a Skin or Scalp Reaction (*LCR*)

1—Extremely rare
2—Rare
3—Average—few reports of problems
4—Higher likelihood of reaction or allergy, depending on the
    level used
5—Avoid

Notice that we have separated out safety and skin reactions. As an example, many people may have allergies to wheat protein, yet wheat protein is a very "safe" ingredient. An herb may be very "safe" on the skin, but have a tendency to cause irritation in some persons.

Further, recall my earlier focus on concentration. Many ingredients may have a perfectly safe level in products, but may exceed that safe level in others. We have rated them based on *the level most commonly found in personal care products*. For example, natural essential oils, sunscreens, menthol, most preservatives and rubefacients like methyl salicylate, all have a level at which they are not likely to irritate, but they all can be skin irritants at higher levels.

Note also that herbal extracts usually contain an herb in a solvent. The solvent may (or may not be) more of a problem than the herb. For example, an herb in alcohol might be more likely to irritate skin than the same herb in glycerin. We rated the herbs with the most commonly used extraction solvent. Be aware that all alcohol extracts, in high concentration, can increase the likelihood of irritation in leave-on products.

For the herbal extracts, the "notes" column lists uses that are mostly anecdotal in nature. With the exception of a few herbs like echinacea, gingko biloba, chamomile and aloe vera, much of the usage notes are historical uses with little or no scientific studies to support these traditional applications. Different types of extracts can contain very different ingredients, depending on the solvent used, source of the herb, time of day harvested, temperature of extraction and so forth.

Lastly, the hardest part. Remember we are discussing the *single ingredients*. The professional formulation of a LCR 4 (higher likelihood of skin reaction) ingredient may make the product a LCR 2 (much less likely to cause a reaction.) Do not assume you can extrapolate all raw material information to all finished formulas. Sometimes you can, many times you cannot. This is precisely the reason that you must choose a company with the expertise to formulate properly and the willingness to share information with you. *This section will address raw materials at the level (percentage) most commonly found in personal care products* (not in their pure form).

5. Restricted and Prohibited Ingredients

We did not list prohibited or restricted ingredients, as it would be unlikely the reader would find them in an ingredient list. Avoid the following wherever you see them:

Bithionol
Mercury compounds (some uses still approved)
Vinyl Chloride
Halogenated salicylanilides
Zirconium complexes in aerosol products
Chloroform
Hexachlorophene
CFCs (Chlorflurocarbon Propellants)
Methylene chloride
Methyl methacrylate monomer in nail formulas
Many artificial colors have been banned (FD&C Red 2, for example)

6. Errors and Omissions; Guarantee of Accuracy

We apologize in advance for any typos or errors. If you believe we have made an error, or omitted important information, please send your written correction to us along with an explanation and technical reference (if possible) to:

Michael Rutledge
c/o Earth Science, Inc.
475 N. Sheridan Street
Corona, CA 92880, USA

We will correct the next edition. We have done our best to insure the accuracy of all information, but it cannot be warranted or guaranteed and should not be considered as absolute. For example, much of the information concerning herbal extracts is anecdotal in nature, and much of the safety information is strictly opinion. This is intended as a guideline only, as the safety of each formula must be evaluated separately by the reader. We accept no responsibility for its accuracy.

Some of the examples in chapters 1 and 2 are several years old and may have been corrected by time of publication.

Now that we have satisfied the attorneys, the balance of this volume is the Ingredient Dictionary, which you may use as a reference when looking at cosmetic ingredients.

Ingredient Name/INCI Name (Other Names in Parentheses)	Source	Purpose	S	LCR	Notes
A					
a (alpha) - Tocopherol See "Tocopherol"					
Acacia (Gum Arabic, Acacia Catechu, Acacia Senegal or Acacia Dealbata)	V	T, S	1	2	Natural gum thickener from the acacia tree in Africa. Also approved as a food additive.
Acetamide MEA	S	M	3	3	Excellent skin conditioner. Light, liquid humectant for skin care. Also used in hair conditioners and as an antistatic electricity agent. Sometimes used to replace glycerin, because it is light and non-sticky. (A nonionic amide)
Acetone (2-Propanone or Dimethyl Ketone)	V, S	SOL	5	4	Can dry the skin in the concentrations used in nail products, etc. Avoid high concentrations. Use in RO products only. Also highly flammable in high concentrations. Can be obtained from fermentation or by chemical synthesis from isopropanol or propane. Beginning to be used in hair sprays to replace alcohol as it is exempt from air pollution regulations.
Acetylated Lanolin (Lanolin Acetate or Acetyl Ester of Lanolin)	A	M	3	4	Generally, more of an occlusive type nonionic moisturizer due to its very oily nature and tendency to form water repellent films. Made from wool lanolin. Not as likely to irritate as lanolin.
Acetylated Lanolin Alcohol (Acetyl Ester of Lanolin Alcohol)	A	M	2	4	Light, emollient liquid, made from wool lanolin. Suspected to be comedogenic, but this depends on the amount used and the other ingredients in the formulation. Helps the "spreadability" of a formula.
Acrylates/Acrylamide Copolymer	S, P	A	4	4	Hair spray/gel holding resin. The ingredient can contain acrylamide monomer as a by-product. The monomer, in sufficient concentration, is a suspected carcinogen. Only the manufacturer will know, as it is not required on the label.

Ingredient Name/INCI Name (Other Names in Parentheses)	Source	Purpose	S	LCR	Notes
Acrylates/beheneth-25 Methacrylate Copolymer	S	T	3	3-4	Thickener for many types of formulas usually used at 1 - 10%.
Acrylates/C10-30 Alkyl Acrylate Crosspolymer	S	T, S	3	3-4	Used primarily as a viscosity increasing and suspending agent. One supplier promotes it as a benzene-free carbomer. (See "Carbomer")
Agar	V	T, A	1	2	Colloid extracted from marine algae. Forms a gel with water. Also used in some micro-encapsulation technology.
Albumen	A	E, T	1	4	Egg derived, water soluble protein. Often used in masks or astringents. Somewhat similar to soy protein in amino acid distribution. Film-former. Also used to temporarily reduce the appearance of wrinkles. Can also be derived from bovine (cattle) sources.
Alcohol (See individual Alcohols)					A large group of ingredients about which few general statements can be made. They are classified as alcohols by their molecular structure and range from the lighter, more drying ethanol, methanol, and isopropanol to solid emollient materials such as cetyl or stearyl alcohol, to the more complex types such as glycerin.
Alcohol denat					New labeling name for denatured ethanol (See "SD Alcohol")
Algae Extract (Various species including Laminaria, Cytoserum, etc.)	V	M, A	1	2	Various strains available for multiple benefits. The polysaccharide content is believed responsible for the unique moisturizing ability. Typically used at 1 - 5% in the formula for effectiveness. Claimed to help protect collagen in the skin, soothe skin and increase cell turnover.
Algin and Sodium Alginate	V	A, T	1	2	Water soluble colloid extracted from marine algae. Also used in some micro-encapsulation technology. Used for gelling or thickening.

Ingredient Name/INCI Name (Other Names in Parentheses)	Source	Purpose	S	LCR	Notes
Alkyl Methacrylates Crosspolymer	S, P	A, T	3	3-4	
Allantoin (2,5-dioxo-4-imidazolidinyl-urea)	V, S	A	2	1	Usually used at 0.2% and lower; healing agent for skin. Found naturally in comfrey plant, most is now synthesized from uric acid. Non-toxic. Stable from pH 4-9. Cell proliferant; helps clear away dead tissue from wounds. Used on cuts, scrapes, burns, sunburns and chapped lips.
Almond Meal	V	Exf	1	1	Very gentle, mild, exfoliant made from crushed almonds. With all exfoliants, the tradeoff is always between being mild and being effective. Almond meal is also an absorbant.
Almond Oil (Bitter) See "Bitter Almond Oil"					
Almond Oil (Sweet) (Purnus Amygdalus Dulcis)	V	M	1	2	Oil pressed or extracted from almonds, used to provide a more elegant "feel" to creams and lotions and help promote "spreading" of the product. Excellent emollient. Food approved. High in omega-6 linoleic acid and other unsaturated fatty acids.
Aloe Barbadensis Gel (Aloe Vera Extract or Juice)	V	M, A	1	2-3	Many types available. Could be fresh juice, an extract, or a concentrate reconstituted with water. The fresh juice is far superior, but the label will not normally tell you which has been used. You are relying solely on the integrity of the manufacturer. Some extracts are mostly ineffective or are used at too low a concentration to perform the intended function. Excellent moisturizer and healing agent when the proper extract is used at sufficient concentrations.
(Aloe Vera) See "Aloe Barbadensis Gel"					

Ingredient Name/INCI Name (Other Names in Parentheses)	Source	Purpose	S	LCR	Notes
Alpha Hydroxy Acids (AHA's)	V, S	A, Exf	3 RO 3-5 LV, Depending on concentration	3 RO 3-5 LV, Depending on concentration	This is a large class of acids. Examples are glycolic acid, lactic acid, tartaric acid and malic acid; used to exfoliate, moisturize and help remove brown spots. They can reduce the appearance of wrinkles when used in a concentration of >5% and a pH below 5. Can also reduce/remove dark spots when used at sufficient concentration. A recent FDA study indicated that they increase UV sensitivity. Fortunately, this seems reversible after discontinuing use of AHAs. For safety, use concentrations below 10% and above pH 3.5. Avoid the sun or use with sunscreens if you must be outdoors. Test these products on a small area of skin before using on a larger portion of your body. Follow directions carefully. Use of high AHA products as exfoliants can make your skin more sensitive to the sun.
Alpha Lipoic Acid (a-Lipoic Acid) AKA Thioctic Acid	V	A	1	1	Powerful, important antioxidant used to neutralize harmful free radicals. It is a synergistic antioxidant, important to maximize the effectiveness of other antioxidants and believed important in the anti-ageing process. Usually a 50-50 blend of two isomers, sometimes called thioctic acid. Its original approved use was to treat Amantia mushroom poisoning.
Althea Extract (Marshmallow Root, or Althea Officinalis)	V	A	2	2	Demulcent (skin soothing agent). Said to promote healing of wounds and cuts. Used as a treatment for bee stings, as a skin softener and emollient.
Alum (Potassium Aluminum Sulfate)	M	A	3 RO 4 LV	3 RO 3-4 LV (At < 0.5%) 5 LV (At > 0.5%)	Astringent, or used as an antiperspirant in deodorant products, such as deodorant stones. Often claimed to be "aluminum-free." That is not correct.
Aluminum Chlorohydrate	M	A	4-5	5	Antiperspirant active ingredient. Commonly used in many commercial products. Believed to work by diffusing into the eccrine sweat ducts, hydrolyzing, then precipitating to form a gel that plugs the sweat ducts. (There are other theories.)

Ingredient Name/INCI Name (Other Names in Parentheses)	Source	Purpose	S	LCR	Notes
Aluminum Tristearate	M,V	T	4	4	Gellant and thickener
Amino Acids (Large group of different ingredients. Look under the individual amino acids for more information.)					The body's building blocks from which all proteins are constructed. They are widely used in skincare to help condition and "moisturize" the skin, and in hair care to act as a hair conditioner.
(Aminobenzoic Acid) See "PABA"					
Aminomethyl Propanol (AMP)	S	pH, SOL	3	3	Neutralizer; solubilizer. A mildly alkaline material used to neutralize the pH of an overly acidic solution, or to neutralize resins and thickeners.
Aminophylline	S	A	2	3-4 Depending on concentration	Anti-cellulite active; works by stimulating blood circulation in the applied area. Vascular dilator, claimed to help open capillaries to help carry waste products away from the area.
Ammonium Chloride	M, S	T	3	3	An electrolyte used to thicken shampoos and cleansers by increasing the ionic strength of the solution. Usually used at less than 1% in formulas.
Ammonium Laureth Sulfate (Ammonium Laureth - 2, 5, 7 or 12 Sulfate) (as the ethoxylation number (2, 5, 7 or 12) increases, mildness increases, and foam and viscosity decrease.)	V	CL	3 RO	3 RO	Cleanser; more mild than ammonium lauryl sulfate. (In general, the laureth form is more mild than the lauryl form.) Used in shampoos and bath gels. (An ethoxylated lauryl alcohol is used in the production instead of lauryl alcohol as in ammonium lauryl sulfate.) Anionic surfactant.

Ingredient Name/INCI Name (Other Names in Parentheses)	Source	Purpose	S	LCR	Notes
Ammonium Lauryl Sulfate	V	CL	3 RO	3-4 RO 4 LV	As with all the cleansers, the mildness rating depends on concentration. Milder than sodium lauryl sulfate (SLS), it is typically made from lauryl alcohol derived from coconut oil. It can be produced by other means. Excellent foamer. The pH must be kept acidic for stability. More stable than SLS at acidic pH. Anionic surfactant.
Ammonium Myreth Sulfate	V	CL	3	3	Mild cleansing, anionic surfactant from myristyl alcohol.
Ammonium Thioglycolate	S	A	4	5	See "Thioglycolic Acid"
Amodimethicone	M	M, A	2	3	Silicone polymer of linked amino acids. Used to improve hair combing and manageability. A reaction product made from dimethicone and an amino type ingredient. This is done to improve functionality in shampoos, and durability on the hair.
Animal Keratin Amino Acids and Animal Collagen Amino Acids	A	M, A	2	3	See "Keratin Amino Acids" or "Hydrolyzed Animal Protein" (Keratin comes only from animals.)
Annatto Extract	V	C	1	1	Delicate, yellow to orange, natural colorant; from plant seeds. Difficult to formulate to achieve a stable color. Tends to fade over time as it ages.
(Antioxidants)					A large class of materials whose function in the body is to neutralize excess "free radicals" resulting from oxidation reactions. It is believed that these free radicals contribute to the ageing process. Some antioxidants are also formulated into products to retard spoilage of the product via oxidation.
Apple Cider Vinegar	V	A, pH	2	3	Mildly acidic astringent; helps reduce sebum flow. Vinegars contain the organic acid – acetic acid, which helps keep the pH low, and thereby can tighten the hair cuticles or neutralize alkaline products.
Apple Extract (Pyrus Malus)	V	A, F	2	2 RO 4 LV	Can be a source of alpha hydroxy acids if extracted properly. The label will not always inform you of the intended use or type of extract.

111

Ingredient Name/INCI Name (Other Names in Parentheses)	Source	Purpose	S	LCR	Notes
Apricot Kernel Oil (Persic Oil, Prunus Armeniaca)	V	M	1	2	Pressed or extracted from apricot seeds, used as a "moisturizer," skin softener and lubricant in skin care. Absorbs into the skin very well. Excellent, light, non-irritating, natural emollient and body oil. High in linoleic acid.
Apricot Seeds (Prunus Armeniaca)	V	Exf	1	2	Crushed seeds of apricots. A source of laetril, if extracted properly. Excellent exfoliant - softer than pumice, more effective than almond meal. Source of emollient apricot kernel oil.
Arbutin	V	A	3	3	Tyrosinase inhibitor. Produces a gradual whitening of the skin by preventing melanin formation. Usually from the leaves of bearberry.
Aristolochia Extract (Aristolochia Fangchi)	V	A	5	3	Herbal extract; suspected carcinogen due to aristolochic acid content.
Arnica Extract (Arnica Montana)	V	A	3 (externally) 5 (internally)	3-4	Anti-irritant, anti-inflammatory and scalp simulator. Has some antiseptic properties. Stimulates blood circulation. Used to treat bruises and aches. Not to be taken internally. Do not apply to broken skin.
Ascorbic Acid (Vitamin C)	V (Dextrose or Glucose micro-biological fermen-tation)	A, O	2	2-4 Depending on concentration	Antioxidant; beta hydroxy acid. Used in the prophylaxis and treatment of photoageing and skin disorders. Important in the anti-ageing process as an antioxidant. Difficult to formulate and maintain stability. Products can turn brown if improperly formulated. Promotes collagen synthesis and can inhibit melanin formation in the skin. Improves performance of sunscreens and provides UV protection for the skin. There is a wide variety of claims being made about vitamin C creams - some of them with little or no scientific support for topical application of vitamin C. Also note that ascorbic acid is very unstable in water-based creams, as it easily oxidizes.
Ascorbyl Glucoside	V	A	2	3	Prepared from ascorbic acid and glucose. A more stable form of ascorbic acid.

Ingredient Name/INCI Name (Other Names in Parentheses)	Source	Purpose	S	LCR	Notes
Ascorbyl Palmitate	V or S	0	2	2	Antioxidant; more stable source of vitamin C (ascorbic acid) in aqueous solutions. Approved for food use. An oil soluble ester of ascorbic acid; more effective than BHA or BHT in preventing rancidity of vegetable oils. One gram = 0.425 grams of ascorbic acid. (The ester of ascorbic acid and palmitic acid)
Astaxanthin	V	0	1-2	2	Multi-purpose antioxidant; an "xanthophyll," member of the carotenoid family. Not water-soluble. Claimed to be an anti-inflammatory, an anti-irritant, and useful in boosting the immune system. Extracted from microalgae and red yeast.
Avobenzone (Parsol 1789, See "Butyl Methoxydibenzoylmethane")					
Avocado Oil (Persea Gratissima)	V	M	1	3	Pressed or extracted from avocados; a vitamin rich oil often used to soften skin. Each fruit or vegetable oil has a different ratio of fatty acids, giving them each unique characteristics. (See Avocado Oil; appendix B) Avocado oil has a lighter "feel" and penetrates the top layers of skin well. Has some UV absorption characteristics.
Awapuhi (Hawaiian Ginger, White Ginger, Hedychium Coronarium	V	M, A	2	2	A moisturizer, believed to have astringent, anti-irritant properties. Used in hair care to lubricate and increase shine.
Azelaic Acid	V	A	3	4	Used as an anti-acne ingredient (a dicarbonic acid made from a fatty acid in castor oil).
Azulene (Guaiazulene)	V	A, C	2	1	Excellent anti-irritant; from German chamomile. Also provides a natural blue to green color, depending on the pH. Can help reduce the overall likelihood of a formula to cause irritation.

Ingredient Name/INCI Name (Other Names in Parentheses)	Source	Purpose	S	LCR	Notes
B					
Babassu Oil (Orbignya Oleifera)	V	M	2	3	Lubricant and good moisturizer; melts close to body temperature; often used in sunscreens in place of coconut oil.
(Baking Soda) See "Sodium Bicarbonate"					
Balm Mint Extract (Lemon Balm or Bee Balm, Melissa Officinalis)	V	A, F	2	3	Skin soother. The essential oil is also used as a fragrance. Also used in cleansers as an acne treatment. Believed to help heal wounds. Tonic; antiseptic.
Balsam (Myroxylon Balsamun, Myroxylon Pereirae)	V	F, A	3	3-4 RO 4 - 5 LV, Depending on concentration	A mixture of resins and fatty acids from various evergreens, shrubs and trees. Usually used in perfumes or as a hair conditioner. Has antiseptic, anti-itch and fungicidal properties. In too high a concentration, it can be an irritant.
Bamboo Oil (Bambusa Vulgaris, Bambusa Arundinacea)	V	P, M	3	3	One extract is used as a preservative. Some bamboo extracts are claimed to function as emollients/moisturizers, others as exfoliants, depending on what type of extract is used.
Basil Extract (Ocimum Basilicum)	V	F, A	2	3	Essential oil used for fragrance component and tonic effect. Used for antibacterial effect in skin healing compounds and as a remedy for digestive complaints and insect stings.
Bearberry Extract (Arctostaphylos Uva-Ursi)	V	A	3	3	Skin lightener; age spot lightener. Contains tannins and the active ingredient arbutin, a natural precursor of hydroquinone. Also has antiseptic and astringent properties. Contrary to its name, usually the dried leaves are used to make the extract. Also used in some oily and acne-prone skin formulas.

Ingredient Name/INCI Name (Other Names in Parentheses)	Source	Purpose	S	LCR	Notes
Bee Pollen	A	A	1	3	The microscopic male seed in flowering plants, collected by bees. Has anti-microbial activity. Rich in amino acids, minerals and some vitamins. There are some reports of pollen allergic reactions.
Beeswax	A	E, T, S	1	2-3	Natural wax collected from beehives, used to help emulsify creams and lotions. Usually used with borax, which reacts with the fatty acids in beeswax, forming sodium salts and a more stable product. Available as bleached or unbleached. There are some reports of pollen allergic reactions.
Behenyl Alcohol (Docosanol)	V	E, M	2	2	Usually made from natural behenic acid, it is a mild solid alcohol, used as an emulsifier, emollient and thickener. (The longer the carbon chain, the higher the viscosity of the finished product, when using fatty alcohols.)
Behentrimonium Chloride	V, S	A	3	3-4	Hair Conditioner; "Quat" type.
Behenyl Behenate	V	T, E	3	3	Emulsifier and viscosity builder in creams and lotions. Non-comedogenic. Can be used to adjust hardness in lipsticks.
Bentonite	M	A, T, S	2	2	Natural silicate colloidal clay to thicken/stabilize products and/or absorb and remove impurities from the skin. Sometimes used as a suspending agent for other ingredients. Excellent in facial masks or acne products to deep clean pores. Very good absorbent. Soothing to the skin – has been used in wound healing.
Benzalkonium Chloride (Alkyl Dimethyl Benzyl Ammonium Chloride)	S	P, A	4-5	4	Antibacterial; topical cationic "Quat" antiseptic incompatible with anionic cleansing surfactants. Avoid eye area - possible eye irritant at higher levels. OTC topical antimicrobial ingredient. Very effective against staphylococcus.
Benzethonium Chloride	S	P, A	4	4	Antiseptic; preservative; cationic "Quat" surfactant
Benzocaine (Ethyl aminobenzoate or; 4-aminobenzoic acid ethyl ester)	S	A	3	3-4	Topical anesthetic; numbing agent. Benzocaine can be a sensitizer in some persons.

Ingredient Name/INCI Name (Other Names in Parentheses)	Source	Purpose	S	LCR	Notes
Benzoic Acid (Phenylformic Acid)	V, S	P	3	3	This and its sodium salt, sodium benzoate, are used as preservatives. Can be derived from gum benzoin. Food approved preservative. Usually used at about 0.1%.
Benzoin (Benzoin Gum, Styrax Benzoin)	V	P	3	4	Natural source of benzoic acid. Also used to "fix" the fragrance in perfume and body products.
Benzophenone-3 and Benzophenone-4 (Oxybenzone) and (Sulisobenzone)	S	A	3	3-4	Sunscreens - more effective than most sunscreens against UVA. Can also be used at low levels (0.1% or less) to protect the color in a product from photo degradation (light destruction). Usually used with other sunscreens to achieve a higher SPF value and broader UV spectrum coverage.
Benzoyl Peroxide	S	A	4	5	Topical antiseptic and drying agent for acne. High likelihood of skin reaction.
Benzyl Alcohol	V, S	F, P, A, SOL	3-4	3	Antibacterial. Can provide a slight numbing effect. Occurs naturally in many essential oils such as jasmine, ylang-ylang and balsam. Also used as a solvent, as a component of fragrances, and for relief of insect bites.
Beta-Carotene	V, S	O, A	1	1	Powerful antioxidant of the carotene family. Helps improve the effectiveness of sunscreens besides being important in the anti-ageing process. (Will make the product yellow at sufficient effective levels.) Sources include algae, vegetables and palm fruit. Can also be made as a corn fermentation product with the fungus, B. Trispora.

Ingredient Name/INCI Name (Other Names in Parentheses)	Source	Purpose	S	LCR	Notes
Betaglucan (Beta Glucan, B-Glucan, Beta 1, 3 Glucan)	V	A	2	2	Derived from the cell walls of yeast or oats, it is an exceptional anti-irritant. It is also believed to be a stimulator of the immune system and help stimulate collagen and elastin production in the skin. Also has film forming and UV protection characteristics. Helps stimulate cell turnover on the skin. It is a hydrocolloid polysaccharide gum, related to guar, carrageenan, pectin and xanthan gum. Also used in wound healing, as an anti-irritant, and as a wrinkle smoother. Important to good skin health.
Beta Hydroxy Acids (BHA's)	V, S	A, M, Exf	3 RO 4 LV	3 RO 4 LV	Similar to alpha hydroxy acids in function and performance. Examples are salicylic acid and benzoic acid. (See "Alpha Hydroxy Acids")
Bergamot Oil (Citrus Aurantium Bergamia)	V	F	3	4	Used in fragrance blends or as a pure aromatherapy oil.
BHA (Butylated Hydroxyanisole)	S	O	5	3	Antioxidant to prevent rancidity (oxidation) of oily substances. Listed as "reasonably anticipated to be (a) human carcinogen in the National Toxicology Program."
BHT (Butylated Hydroxytoluene)	S	O	4	3	Antioxidant to prevent rancidity (oxidation) of oily substances.
Bilberry Extract (Vaccinium Myrtillus)	V	A	2	3	Antioxidant; astringent (contains tannins); mild antiseptic. Anthocyanosides and glycosides are active ingredient groups. Believed to contribute to capillary health to a greater degree than bioflavonoids. Commonly used to assist in relief of eye fatigue and reduction of eye irritation. Internally, it has been used to support optimum eye health, protect vision and improve night vision. (From the berries.)

Ingredient Name/INCI Name (Other Names in Parentheses)	Source	Purpose	S	LCR	Notes
Bioflavonoids	V	A	1	2	Large group of ingredients from plants used as antioxidants in anti-aging products. Believed to stimulate collagen production in the skin. Also valuable for a variety of internal body processes and preventative for many disorders. Believed to contribute to capillary health and inhibit blood clot formation. Generally, they also have anti-inflammatory properties via their anti-oxidant action and via lipoxygenase (an enzyme) inhibition. They have high reactivity and can "bind" heavy metal ions in the body. Grape seed, green tea, ginkgo and some citrus extracts are all good sources of bioflavonoids.
Biotin (Vitamin H, Coenzyme R)	V, A, S	A	2	2	Used at very low concentrations. Growth factor, present in every living cell. Also used to add body or shine to hair care formulas. Some believe it to assist in hair growth from the scalp. Ability to grow hair on the scalp is unproven. Commonly used in hair and nail preparations to encourage growth. Internally used for a variety of metabolism functions, including seborrheic dandruff and acne. A deficiency can lead to dermatitis. One source is derived from yeast.
Birch Bark Extract (Betula Alba, White Birch)	V	A	2	3	Astringent; hair conditioner; tonic for skin and scalp. High methyl salicylate content. Sometimes used on dark spots or freckles to help lighten them. Has anti-inflammatory and antiseptic properties. Active ingredients are betulin and betulinic acid.
Bisabolol (a-Bisabolol)	V	A	2	1	Anti-irritant; anti-microbial from chamomile. Anti-inflammatory active of chamomile. Used in wound healing. Also extracted from a South American tree - vanillosmopsis erythropappa.
Bismuth Oxychloride	M	C	3	3	Pearlescent pigment or filler; usually used in powders. Improves skin adhesion of powders.
Bitter Almond Oil (Prunus Amygdalus Amara)	V	M	2	3-5	Primary component is benzaldahyde. The aromatic essential oils from almond oil; also used as a flavor.

Ingredient Name/INCI Name (Other Names in Parentheses)	Source	Purpose	S	LCR	Notes
Black Cohosh Extract (Cimicifuga Racemosa)	V	A	3	3	Astringent. Typically used for its estrogenic effect in women's products. The roots are normally used in producing the extract. An active ingredient is triterpenoid glycosides (27-deoxyacteine). Also has anti-inflammatory and antibiotic properties. Contains phytoestrogens; used internally in the treatment of female menopause.
Black Currant Oil (Ribes Nigrum)	V	A	2	3	Excellent emollient and source of essential fatty acids. High in oleic, linoleic and linolenic acids. (A source of omega-3 and omega-6 fatty acids)
Bladderwrack Extract (Kelp, Fucus Vesiculosus)	V	A	2	2	(See Seaweed Extract)
Borage Oil (Borago Officinalis)	V	M, A	3	3	Rich in omega-6 fatty acids and one of the best sources of gamma linolenic acid (25-30%) and other emollient fatty acids. Helps repair/restore the intracellular moisture barrier of the skin. The aqueous extract of borage contains allantoin and is an anti-irritant. From the flowering tops and leaves. Linoleic acid content is about 35-40%.
(Borax) See "Sodium Borate"					
Boric Acid	M	P, A, pH	3-4 (External Use) 5 (Internal Use)	4	Used as a preservative; pH adjuster; antibacterial. The sodium salt of boric acid is sodium borate (or borax). Larger amounts of Boric Acid (well above preservative level) can be a risk for internal poisoning. For this reason it is prohibited in baby powders. It is considered relatively harmless if properly used at low levels externally.
Brassica Campestris/Aleurites Fordi Oil Copolymer	V	A, M	3	3	A polymer made via pressurized steam in a low oxygen atmosphere from china wood oil and canola oil. Used as a moisturizer and film former to aid in increasing water resistance and shine.

Ingredient Name/INCI Name (Other Names in Parentheses)	Source	Purpose	S	LCR	Notes
Bromelain	V	A	2	3-4	Enzyme from pineapples. Used in light skin peels to help exfoliate the skin. Concentration is very important to effectiveness.
2-Bromo-2 Nitropropane - 1, 3-Diol	S	P	4	5	Preservative; believed to work by providing formaldehyde in the product. Anti-bacterial; antifungal. Can form nitrosamines (carcinogens) when combined with certain amines or amides, under certain conditions.
Burdock Root Extract (Arctium Majus or Arctium Lappa)	V	A	3	3	Eczema, psoriasis and acne treatment; anti-itch remedy. Oily skin treatment. Has antibacterial properties. Used as a dandruff treatment in some formulas.
Butyl Alcohol (n-Butyl Alcohol, Butanol)	S	SOL	4	4	Solvent
Butylene Glycol (1, 3-Butylene Glycol)	S	M	3	3	Solvent, often used to replace propylene glycol. Believed to be less likely to cause a skin reaction than propylene glycol. Also has preservative properties at concentrations above about 15%. Produced from a reaction between acetaldehyde and sodium hydroxide.
Butyl Ester of PVP/MA Copolymer	S	A	3	3	Polymer used to coat the hair and hold it in place. More flexible than some of the other common resins. Usually neutralized with aminomethyl propanol or some other alkaline material, to increase water solubility.
Butyl Methoxydibenzoylmethane (Avobenzone)	S	A	3	3 - 4	Primarily a UVA sunscreen, but also provides UVB protection. Normally used in combinations with UVB sunscreens to provide broad spectrum UVA/UVB protection. Can be used to protect the products themselves from light degradation. Not compatible with PABA and PABA esters.
Butylparaben (4-Hydroxybenzoic acid butyl ester)	S	P	4	4	Oil soluble preservative, typically used at 0.2% and less, and in combination with other preservatives to achieve broader spectrum coverage. The only paraben soluble in hydrocarbons. Not a formaldehyde donor as are many preservatives.

C

Ingredient Name/INCI Name (Other Names in Parentheses)	Source	Purpose	S	LCR	Notes
C18-36 Acid Triglyceride	V	E, M, T, S	2	2	Excellent emulsifier and can provide rigidity in stick products due to its wax-like characteristics. Also used as a moisturizer and emulsion stabilizer. Some similarities in performance to carnauba wax.
C12-15 Alkyl Benzoate (C12-15 Alcohol Benzoate)	S	M	3	2	Emollient ester used to make "oily" products less oily feeling. Provides a more "dry" feel to the formula. Helps solubilize some difficult-to-solubilize materials such as sunscreens and silicones. Low toxicity; non-comedogenic.
C14-16 Olefin Sulfonates (AOS, Alpha Olefin sulfonates)	S, P	CI	3	4	High foaming cleansers, even in hard water or with oily hair.
Calcium Ascorbate	V, S	A	2	3-4	Stable, non-acidic form of vitamin C
Calcium Carbonate (Chalk)	M	AB	2	2	Typically used as an abrasive in toothpaste. Also used in powders as an absorbant. Tends to make powders "dry" feeling.
Calcium Lactate	M, V	M	3	3	The calcium salt of lactic acid; good humectant properties. Use level about 2-5%.
Calcium Panthothenate	S	A	2	2	Source of pantothenic acid (B-vitamin). Used as a hair conditioner also. Has some humectant properties. It is the calcium salt of the "d" isomer of pantothenic acid.
Calendula Extract (Calendula Officinalis)	V	A	3	3	Anti-inflammatory; wound healer; used on rashes, burns, insect stings, etc. Used in general healing ointments. Has antiseptic properties.
Camphor (Cinnamomum Camphora)	V	A, P	3 (External Use)	3-4	Natural camphor is used as a topical antibacterial. It has a pungent, characteristic odor. From the camphor tree; can be synthesized. Provides a warming, then cooling sensation on the skin. Also has anti-inflammatory effects and astringent properties. Excellent at low levels. Do not ingest. Do not use synthetic "camphorated oil" which has a high toxicity.

Ingredient Name/INCI Name (Other Names in Parentheses)	Source	Purpose	S	LCR	Notes
Canadian Willowherb Extract (Epilobium Angustifolium)	V	A	2	2	Used as an aid in wound-healing and as an anti-inflammatory. Has anti-irritant and antioxidant properties. Contains a variety of active ingredients, including proanthocyandins.
Candelilla Wax (Euphorbia Cerifera)	V	T	2	3	Natural wax, used primarily for hardening stick type products. Provides hardness, rigidity and gloss to lipsticks.
Cannabis Sativa Seed Oil (Hempseed Oil)	V	M	3	3	Fatty acid oil; source of linoleic acid and other fatty acids from the hemp plant.
Canolamidopropyl Betaine	V	CL	3	2-3	A mild amphoteric type cleanser made from canola oil
Canola Oil (Rapeseed Oil)	V	M	1	3	Emollient, lubricant, provides "slip" to creams and lotions. Linoleic acid content is about 20-30%. Alpha linolenic content is about 7-15%.
Capryl/Capramido Betaine	V	CL	3	2-3	A mild amphoteric type cleanser
Caprylic/Capric Triglyceride	V	M	2	3	Excellent moisturizer, emollient and solubilizer. Has lubricant properties also. Also used as a solvent for perfume ingredients and flavors. (A triglyceride of fatty acids.) Non-greasy.
Capsaicin (Capsicum Oleoresin, Capsicum Frutescens)	V	A	3	4-5	Natural cayenne pepper extract used to create "heat" in muscle/joint pain treatments. Too much, or the wrong extract, can harm the skin. Concentration is crucial. Works by blocking the pain neurotransmitters. Stimulates circulation. One of a very few ingredients intentionally formulated to produce a skin reaction.
Captan	S	A, P	4	5	Fungicide: bacteriostat
Caramel	V	C	1	1	Colorant made from heating sugar or corn syrup. Approved for food use.

Ingredient Name/INCI Name (Other Names in Parentheses)	Source	Purpose	S	LCR	Notes
Carbomer (Common Trade Name "Carbopol®," Acrylic Acid Polymer)	S	T, S	3	3-5	There is a series of these high molecular weight polymers of acrylic acid. In and of themselves, they are not harmful, but one should avoid those with high benzene levels. The label will not indicate which ones have such a level. Check with your manufacturer. Carbomers are thickening and gelling agents which can provide a clear, stable gel. The European standard, for example, sets a limit of 1,000 ppm benzene for cosmetics and 2ppm for drugs. There are some grades available using ethyl acetate and cyclohexane instead of benzene. (See "Acrylates C10-30 Alkyl Acrylate Crosspolymer")
Carboxymethyl Cellulose (CMC) or Sodium Carboxymethyl Cellulose or Cellulose Gum (CTFA name)	V	T, S	2	2	Thickener, stabilizer and suspending agent, stable between about pH 5.5 - 9.5. If pure, essentially an inert, cellulose derivative. Some pharmaceutical and food uses approved.
Carmine (Cochineal, Carminic Acid)	A	C	2	2	Natural color. Red pigment extracted from the hard exoskeleton of cochineal, a Latin-American insect. Used for thousands of years in many cultures. Approved for food use. The color material extracted is carminic acid. Can also be in the form of the sodium or ammonium salt, or the "lake" color. See "lake" in "terms" section.
Carnauba Wax (Copernicia Cerifera)	V	T, S	2	2	Generally used in sticks (like lipsticks) to harden the stick to the proper consistency. Also used to raise the melting point. (A naturally occurring wax.) From leaves and buds of the carnauba palm. Can be formed into spheres and used as an exfoliant.
(Carob Bean Gum) See "Locust Bean Gum"					

Ingredient Name/INCI Name (Other Names in Parentheses)	Source	Purpose	S	LCR	Notes
(Carotene) See "Beta-Carotene"					Beta-Carotene is the most commonly used of the carotene group of anti-oxidants. (Carotenoids)
Carrageenan (Chondrus Crispus)	V	T, S	2	2	Natural thickener and gel forming gum polysaccharide from various seaweeds and algaes. Helps stabilize formulas or suspend various ingredients. Usually from red seaweeds (see Irish Moss). Also used as an emollient to counteract dry skin and hair.
Carrot Oil (Daucus Carota)	V	A, M, C	1	1	Used as a source of beta-carotene and as a safe, natural coloring agent. Approved for food use.
Castor Oil (Oil of Palma Christi, Ricinus Communis)	V	M, SOL	4	3	High viscosity oil. From the castor bean. Used commonly in lipsticks to help suspend the pigments and produce a good film on the lips. Excellent barrier agent (occlusive) and emollient. The seeds of the plant are poisonous. Use only a properly manufactured oil. Also used to help disperse the pigments in lipsticks and other colored products.
Cat's Claw Extract (Uncaria Tomentosa, Una de gato)	V	A	3	3	A rainforest herb used in Peru to treat a variety of ailments, including arthritis, infections and ulcers. The quinovic acid glycosides in cat's claw have anti-inflammatory properties. Also reported to have immune-enhancing effects. Used in the treatment of cancer and AIDS in some studies. As with all herbs it is important to select the right extract with the correct active ingredients. There are two types of *U.tomentosa* - one more biologically active than the other. Also has antioxidant and anti-mutagenic properties. [One of the anti-inflammatory active groups is called pentacyclic oxindole alkaloids (POA)].
Cedar Oil or Cedar Extract (Thuja Occidentalis)	V	F	3-4	3-5 Depending on concentration	Fragrance. Also used as an insect repellant. The pure oil, from the cedar tree, by itself can be irritating. At low levels in a fragrance, there is less likelihood. Other extracts can have astringent properties.

Ingredient Name/INCI Name (Other Names in Parentheses)	Source	Purpose	S	LCR	Notes
Cellulose Gum (made from Cellulose)	V	T, S	1	1	A sugar based polymer, typically used to thicken products. Cellulose is part of the cell wall and structural component of plants, and one of the most abundant naturally occurring organic substances. Cellulose is a polysaccharide. Also used as an absorbant. (See Carboxymethylcellulose)
Centella Asiatica (See Gotu Kola Extract)					The extract usually contains asiaticoside, madecassic acid and asiatic acid (from the leaves).
Ceramides 1, 2, 3, 4, 33, etc. (Ceramides are a large group of ingredients)	V, A, S	M, A	2	2-3	They mimic the intercellular lipids in our own skin, promoting healthy moisturization and supple skin. Some, (not all) ceramides are a natural part of your skin. They are also skin conditioners and contribute to the skin's moisture barrier. Many are animal derived. Studies indicate that as we age, the amount of ceramides in the skin decreases. (See "Sunflower Seed Extract")
Ceresin Wax	M, S	T, S	3	3	Used to help raise the melting point and increase stiffness in stick products. Contains ozokerite and other waxes. Sometimes it is a name given to a type of ozokerite wax (See Ozokerite), produced by refining and bleaching.
Ceteareth-4, -5, -6, -7, -8, -9, -10, -12, -20, etc.	V	E	2	3	Emulsifiers for creams and lotions, made from fatty acid alcohols, primarily cetyl and stearyl.
Cetearyl Alcohol	V	E, M, T	2	2	Mixture of cetyl and stearyl alcohol. Forms dense emulsions. Also used as a thickener and emollient.
Cetearyl Glucoside	V	E	2	2	Sugar-based emulsifier
Cetearyl Octanoate	V	E, M	2	3	Emollient; emulsifier; promotes quick spreading of the formula. In hair products, produces gloss and sheen. (A clear, colorless liquid)
Cetearyl Palmitate	V	E, M	2	3	Emollient; emulsifier

Ingredient Name/INCI Name (Other Names in Parentheses)	Source	Purpose	S	LCR	Notes
Ceteth - 5, -10, -20, etc.	V, S	E	2	3	Non-ionic emulsifiers for creams and lotions. Formed from cetyl alcohol and a PEG polymer.
Cetrimonium Bromide	V, S	A	3	3 RO 4 LV	Antistatic electricity hair conditioner; antiseptic; cationic surfactant
Cetrimonium Chloride	V, S	A	3	3 RO 4 LV	Antistatic electricity hair conditioner; antiseptic; cationic surfactant
Cetrimonium Silicone Carboxy Complex	M	A	3	3 RO 3 LV	Good skin conditioner. Soothes and conditions skin to help prevent dry skin. Anti-irritant. Can reduce oiliness. Less likely to irritate than cetrimonium bromide or chloride because of the silicone. (A combination of a "Quat" and a silicone)
Cetyl Alcohol	V	E, M, T	2	2	White, slightly waxy solid material, usually used as an aid to emulsification in creams and lotions. (Not a "drying" alcohol.) Produces a more "dense" emulsion. Approved for use in pharmaceuticals. (From vegetable oils but it can be synthesized also.)
Cetyl Dimethicone (Alkyl Modified Silicone)	M, S	M	3	3	A derivative of dimethicone, that can produce a thicker final product and/or improved skin feel and "spreadability" vs. dimethicone. (See "Dimethicone")
Cetyl Esters	V	E	2	3	Excellent nonionic emulsifier and lubricant; imparts "body" to emulsions and improves stability. A.K.A. Synthetic spermaceti wax - used to replace the whale derived product. Can be used as a thickener also. (A mixture of saturated fatty acids and fatty alcohols)
Cetyl Octanoate	V	E, M	2	3	Wetting agent; helps spreadability of the formula. Emollient.
Cetyl Palmitate	V	E, M	2	3	Produces a more viscous emulsion than cetearyl palmitate. Also has emollient properties as it has a "waxy" consistency. The ester of cetyl alcohol and palmitic acid.
Cetyl Phosphate	V, M, S	E, M	3	3	Made by the reaction of cetyl alcohol and phosphoric acid.

Ingredient Name/INCI Name (Other Names in Parentheses)	Source	Purpose	S	LCR	Notes
Chamomile Extract (Matricaria Extract, Chamomilla Recutita -German Chamomile, Anthemis Nobilis - Roman or English Chamomile)	V	A	2	3	Used as an anti-irritant, anti-swelling agent and tonic in skin care. In hair care, used to bring forth natural highlights of the hair. Source of azulene and bisabolol. Anti-inflammatory. Some reports of pollen allergy reactions. There are several types of chamomile and many types of extracts. You must rely completely on your manufacturer to select the correct extract for the intended purpose. Some extracts have a high flavanoid content that is claimed to help broken capillaries. We have not seen this proven in external applications.
Cherry Bark Extract (Prunus Avium)	V	A, F	2	3	Flavor; fragrance; antioxidant. (From the bark of the cherry tree)
Chitosan	A	A	2	3	Derived from chitin, found in the shells of crustaceans. Used as a flexible film former and moisture retention agent. (It is the partially deacetylated derivative of chitin.) Has some anti-bacterial properties. Used in deodorants and as a sunscreen water resistance enhancer.
Chloroxylenol	S	P	4	5	Used as a preservative and occasionally as a topical antibacterial.
Cholecalciferol (Vitamin D)	S, A	A	3	3 (At <0.1%) 4 (At > 0.1%)	Emollient and moisturizer. Enhances performance of vitamin A. Internally used for proper calcium and phosphorous absorption and bone building, normal growth and development, and anti-aging. Prevents rickets. One source is produced from cholesterol.
Cholesterol	A	M, A, E	2	2	Natural component of human sebum (skin oil) and all body tissues, it is believed to help "moisturize" the skin by keeping the skin more supple. Used as a moisturizer and emollient (an animal sterol). Also used as an emulsifier in creams, lotions and ointments. The body makes cholesterol from squalene produced in the sebaceous glands.
Chromium Oxide Green	M	C	4 (External Use) 5 (Internal Use)	4	Natural mineral color

Ingredient Name/INCI Name (Other Names in Parentheses)	Source	Purpose	S	LCR	Notes
Chromium Picolinate	M	A	3-4	4	A source of the essential trace element, chromium. Chromium is bound to the natural substance - picolinic acid in this molecule. This makes it more bioavailable. Also useful in weight loss, controlling blood sugar levels, increasing lean muscle mass, cholesterol control and increasing the effectiveness of insulin. Note that while chromium is an essential human body element, avoid the form "hexavalent chromium" in high concentration as it is a known carcinogen. Important in the metabolism of carbohydrates and fats. Normal daily intake has been recommended as 50-400 mcg. Internally, studies indicate it can also help insulin users increase glucose uptake.
Cinnamon Oil (Cassia Oil, Cinnamomum Cassia, Cinnamomum Zeylanicum)	V	A, F	3	4-5	Used as a flavor or fragrance. Also used to promote circulation in the skin in some cellulite treatment products. Can cause a burning sensation on the skin if improperly formulated. Common allergen. Has antibacterial properties.
Citric Acid	V, S	pH	2	2	Usually used to lower the pH of the formula. Naturally occurring, weak organic acid. Much is prepared via fermentation of molasses by yeasts. Commonly found in citrus fruits.
Citrus Bioflavonoids (See Bioflavonoids)	V				
Citrus Extract	V	A	2	3-4 Depending on which extract is used, and at which concentration	Various extracts are available, and the term can mean several different things. Some extracts can be a source of alpha hydroxy acids. Some oils are a source of d-limonene. Also used as a flavor, fragrance and disinfectant. Orange peel extract for example has anti-inflammatory, antibacterial and antifungal properties.
(Clover Extract) See "Red Clover Leaf Extract"					

Ingredient Name/INCI Name (Other Names in Parentheses)	Source	Purpose	S	LCR	Notes
Coal Tar	M	A	5	4-5	Used in various skin and scalp treatments, and some dandruff shampoos. Listed as a carcinogen in the National Toxicology Program. (From coal)
Cocamide DEA	V	T, CL, E	3-4	3-4	The amides are used to thicken, increase foam, cleanse and to help solubilize other ingredients. Improper formulation combined with free DEA can lead to the formation of nitrosamines, under certain circumstances.
Cocamide MEA	V	T, CL, E	3	3	The uses are similar to those of Cocamide DEA, except it is produced with monoethanolamine (MEA) instead of diethanolamine (DEA). A mixture of ethanolamines of fatty acids. A recent report shows a low toxicity level.
Cocamidopropylamine Oxide	V	CL	3	3	Mild foaming cleanser. Used to increase the foam in some cleansers. Has anti-static properties at low pH. Also used to thicken formulas that contain sulfate type cleansers.
Cocamidopropyl Betaine	V	CL	3	2	Mild foaming amphoteric cleanser
Cocamidopropyl Dimethylamine	V	A	3	3-4	Cationic emulsifier with enhanced substantivity to skin and hair. Lower irritation than normal quaternary conditioners.
Cocamidopropyl Hydroxysultaine	V	CL	3	3	Mild cleansing amphoteric surfactant with hair conditioning properties. Foam booster. Makes alkyl sulfate systems less irritating. Stable at high and low pH.
Cocarboxylase	S, V, A	A	2	2	Easily absorbable, very active, enzyme form of Vitamin B_1
Cocoa Butter (Theobroma Cacao)	V	M	2	3	Excellent occlusive moisturizer and emollient, but relatively "greasy" feeling in higher concentrations. Used to treat sunburn and as a massage lubricant. Melts at body temperature. A natural vegetable fat from the cocoa (or cacao) tree, native to Central and South America. (Do not confuse with Coca shrub or coconut palm.) The cocoa bean is about 50% cocoa butter.

129

Ingredient Name/INCI Name (Other Names in Parentheses)	Source	Purpose	S	LCR	Notes
Cocoamphocarboxyglycinate	V	CL	3	2	Very mild foaming amphoteric cleanser. Prepared from coconut fatty acids through several reaction steps.
Coco-Betaine	V	CL	3	2	Mild, foaming amphoteric cleanser and good foam booster. Has some anti-static properties. Substantive to hair. Cationic in acidic solution; anionic in alkaline solution. Foams well over a wide pH range.
Cocodimonium Hydrolyzed Animal Protein	A	M, A	3	3	An animal protein, "quaternized" for the purpose of increasing the substantivity to hair and skin. (See "Quaternary Ammonium Compound" in the "terms" section.
Coconut Oil (Cocos Nucifera)	V	M	2	2	Moisturizer, commonly found in sunscreen products; high melting oil, solid at room temperature. Derivative compounds, usually with "coco" in the name, make up a large percentage of cosmetic ingredients. Its stability and availability make it an excellent starting point for the manufacturer of many emulsifiers and cleansers. Its fatty acids, particularly lauric and stearic, are used to produce many other ingredients.
Codecarboxylase (Pyridoxal 5'-Phosphate)	S	A	2	3	The more active, enzyme form of vitamin B_6. More bioavailable in the body. Necessary for biotin synthesis.
(Coenzyme A)					The coenzyme form of Pantothenic Acid. (See "Pantothenic Acid".)
Coenzyme Q-10 (Ubiquinone)	A, V, S	A	2	2	Powerful, lipid soluble, anti-ageing antioxidant and cardiovascular agent. One of a series of coenzymes, Q6 - Q10 are naturally occurring in the majority of aerobic organisms, from bacteria to higher plants and animals. Taken internally, noted for its heart protecting effects and prevention of other cardiovascular conditions. In the body, it is largely located in the nucleus, lipoproteins, and mitochondria of cells.

Ingredient Name/INCI Name (Other Names in Parentheses)	Source	Purpose	S	LCR	Notes
Collagen (For Hydrolyzed Collagen, see Hydrolyzed animal protein)	A	A, M	2	2	A protein used to help temporarily moisturize and tighten skin. This is a purely animal derived product. No plant source. One of the major constituents of skin and connective tissue. Denaturing of collagen produces gelatin. (See "Soluble Collagen")
Colloidal Sulfur (See Sulfur)					
Comfrey Extract (Symphytum Officinale)	V	A	3	3	Skin soother; emollient. Used as a wound healer. High allantoin content. Reduces inflammation associated with injury. Safe for use in cosmetics. Do not ingest.
Copper PCA (Copper Pyroglutamate or Copper Pyrrolidone Carboxylic Acid)	M	A	3	3	Antimicrobial and moisturizer. The copper is bound to the PCA molecule (see "Sodium PCA") and is not "free" copper. Claimed to help accelerate tanning because it is important to melanin formation. Copper is an essential trace mineral, important in the body's keratin and collagen production. Helps reduce dandruff on the scalp; typically used at 0.05-0.5%.
Coriander Extract (Coriandrum Sativum)	V	A, F	3	3	The pure oil is used as a fragrance component. Used as an external treatment for rheumatic joints and muscles. Also used in products for digestion.
Cornflower Extract (Centaurea Cyanus) AKA Bluebottle Extract	V	A	2	2	Astringent, tonic, soothing, wound healing. The extract sometimes used for eyewashes, eyedrops, chapped lips and mouth sores.
Cranberry Extract (Vaccinium Macrocarpon)	V	A	1	2-3	Has astringent properties and antibacterial properties. Has been used as a natural acne treatment.
Cranberry Juice (Vaccinium Macrocarpon)	V	A	1	2	Has astringent properties and antibacterial properties. Has been used as a natural acne treatment. The juice is bitter and is usually diluted with water.
(Crushed Apricot Seeds) See "Apricot Seeds"					

Ingredient Name/INCI Name (Other Names in Parentheses)	Source	Purpose	S	LCR	Notes
(Crushed or ground Loofa) See "Luffa Cylindrica"	V	Exf	1	2	Used as an exfoliant in body scrubs
Cucumber Extract (Cucumis Sativus)	V	A	2	2	Skin softener; sometimes used to reduce dark circles under eyes. Also used to help reduce oily skin.
Cyanocobalamin (Vitamin B₁₂)	S, A, V (Usually micro-biological fermen-tation)	A	2	2	Not found in plants – often supplemented by vegetarians. Internally used for normal growth and development, red blood cells, for nerve damage, anemia and used as an AIDS treatment. Good for severe burns or injuries.
Cyclodextrin	V	A	2	2	Often used to coat, adsorb or encapsulate other active ingredients to reduce irritation potential or provide a slower release of the active ingredients.
Cyclomethicone	M, S	M, SOL	3	3	The lightest, non-greasy silicone. Not as effective as a moisture barrier as the other silicones, but more "dry" feeling and less oily feeling.
Cypress Extract (Cupressus Sempervirens)	V	A	2	3	Skin soother; helps reduce dark circles around the eyes; anti-irritant. Vasoconstrictor. Has astringent properties.
Cysteine (L–Cysteine, Cystein)	A, V, S	A	2	3	Amino acid used as a hair and skin conditioner. Also has anti-oxidant properties. Used in hair waving as a mild reducing agent. A product of the oxidation of cystine.
Cystine (Cystin)	A, S	A	2	3	Amino acid constituent of hair, used as a hair conditioner. Used in hair waving as a conditioner.
D					
D&C Blue #4	S	C	4	4	Artificial color. D&C means the FDA has approved it for use in Drugs and Cosmetics (not foods).

Ingredient Name/INCI Name (Other Names in Parentheses)	Source	Purpose	S	LCR	Notes
D&C Brown #1 (Resorcin Brown)	S	C	4	4	Artificial color. D&C means the FDA has approved it for use in Drugs and Cosmetics (not foods).
D&C Green #5 (Alizarine Cyanine Green)	S	C	4	4	Artificial color. D&C means the FDA has approved it for use in Drugs and Cosmetics (not foods).
D&C Orange #5 (Dibromofluoroescein)	S	C	4	4	Artificial color. D&C means the FDA has approved it for use in Drugs and Cosmetics (not foods).
D&C Red #6	S	C	4	4	Artificial color. D&C means the FDA has approved it for use in Drugs and Cosmetics (not foods).
D&C Red #21 (Tetrabromofluoroescein)	S	C	4	4	Artificial color. D&C means the FDA has approved it for use in Drugs and Cosmetics (not foods).
D&C Red #30	S	C	4	4	Artificial color. D&C means the FDA has approved it for use in Drugs and Cosmetics (not foods). (Indigold type)
Ext. D&C Yellow #7 (Napthol Yellow S)	S	C	4	4	Artificial color. D&C means the FDA has approved it for use in Drugs and Cosmetics (not foods). (Xanthene type)
D&C Yellow #8 (Uranine)	S	C	4	4	Artificial color. D&C means the FDA has approved it for use in Drugs and Cosmetics (not foods).
D&C Yellow #10	S	C	4	4	Artificial color. D&C means the FDA has approved it for use in Drugs and Cosmetics (not foods).
Dandelion Extract (Taraxacum Officinale)	V	A	2	3-4	Skin soother and tonic. Internally used as a liver treatment.
DEA (Diethanolamine) ("DEA" can mean "Diethanolamide" when used as a suffix)	S	pH	3-4 RO 4-5 LO (See pages 17-19)	4	Mildly alkaline material used to raise the pH and/or neutralize alkaline substances. Produces a milder surfactant when used in place of sodium hydroxide. (See "DEA Laureth Sulfate," for example.) There is some evidence that it can react with other ingredients to form carcinogens if not properly formulated.

Ingredient Name/INCI Name (Other Names in Parentheses)	Source	Purpose	S	LCR	Notes
DEA-Cetyl Phosphate (Diethanolamine Salt of Cetyl Phosphate)	V, S, M	E	3	3-4	Anionic surfactant, emulsifier and emulsion stabilizer. Made by reacting cetyl alcohol with phosphoric acid, then reacting that product with diethanolamine.
DEA-Laureth Sulfate	V	CL, E	3	3	The "DEA" part of the molecule means that its acidic part has been neutralized with DEA. The amount of "free DEA" left over varies from manufacturer to manufacturer. It is this "free DEA" in DEA neutralized ingredients that causes the most concern. Your manufacturer can solve this problem by the selection of a good supplier and proper formulation.
DEA-Oleth-3, 5, 10, etc. Phosphate	S, M, V	E, T	3	3-4	Anionic emulsifier and thickener. Oil in water emulsifiers for a variety of purposes, including micro-emulsion gels. (A phosphate ester)
Decyl Alcohol (Capric Alcohol)	V, S	E, M	2	2	A fatty acid derived alcohol, commonly used as an emulsifier and/or emollient.
Decyl Cocoate	V	E, M	3	3	Emollient oil with good "spreadability"
Decyl Esters of Olive Oil Extract (Decyl Olivate and Squalene)	V	M	3	3	An emollient oil made from olive oil and squalene
Decyl Glucoside (Decyl Polyglucose)	V	CL	3	2-3	Very mild, nonionic, corn-derived, surfactant cleanser. Does not foam (lather) as well as many other surfactants. (Product of a corn-starch glucose polymer and decyl alcohol)
Decyl Oleate	V, S	M, SOL	3	3	Lubricant, emollient and provides "slip" to various products. Non-tacky. (Ester of decyl alcohol and oleic acid)
Dehydroacetic Acid or Sodium Dehydroacetate	S	A	3-4	3-4 RO 4-5 LV	Fungicide; bactericide
(Deionized Water) See "Water"					"Deionized Water" is not a correct labeling name.

Ingredient Name/INCI Name (Other Names in Parentheses)	Source	Purpose	S	LCR	Notes
Dextran	V	T	2	2	A group of polysaccharides of varying molecular weights. (Fermentation product)
Dextrin	V	E, S, T	1	2	Produced by the partial hydrolysis of starch
DHA (See "Dihydroxyacetone")					Note: "DHA" can also be the abbreviation for an Omega-3 fatty acid from fish oil, known as docosahexaenoic acid. (Not related to dihydroxyacetone)
DHEA (Dehydroepiandosterane)	S	A	3-5 (No long term safety studies)	3	A natural steroid, not really a hormone, but commonly referred to as a "master" hormone because it regulates or helps regulate so many hormonal functions. The amount in our bodies declines with age. Taken internally, it increases the level of androgens and estrogens in the body. Claimed to increase immune function and reduce blood pressure.
Diazolidinyl Urea	S	P	3	3 RO 4-5 LV Depending on use and concentration	Commonly used preservative. While most preservatives are more likely than most other ingredients to be a source of irritation to sensitive persons, they are necessary. This is one of the better preservatives in that regard, in our opinion.
(Dicetyldimonium Chloride) See "Quaternium 31"					
Dicalcium Phosphate	M	AB	3	3	Commonly used as an abrasive in toothpastes. Better taste than calcium carbonate, and lower pH.
Diethylene Glycol	S	M, SOL	5	4	Possible toxic effects if absorbed through the skin
Diglycerin (Diglycerol)	V, S	M, SOL	2	3	Similar to glycerin; not as sticky. Approved for some food use. Good humectant.
Dihydroxyacetone (DHA, or 1, 3-dihydroxy-2-propanone)	V, S	A	3	3-4	Artificial tanning agent that darkens skin without the sun. Works by forming a brown stain via a reaction with certain amino acids of skin keratin. Usually prepared by the fermentation of glycerin; a simple sugar, that is part of the carbohydrate metabolism in higher plants and animals. Generally non-toxic.

Ingredient Name/INCI Name (Other Names in Parentheses)	Source	Purpose	S	LCR	Notes
Dimethicone	M	M	2	2	This is a silicone. Silicones are polymers based on silica (sand) and processed to form different molecules. They are generally inert and non toxic to skin. Widely used in skin and hair care products for emolliency, water proofing, reducing stickiness, improving skin feel, and hair conditioning. Also improves combability of the hair. Because silicones suppress foam, they are occasionally used as anti-foaming agents.
Dimethicone Copolyol	M	M, E	2-3	2-3	Silicone polymer used as a moisturizer, lubricant, shine producer, occlusive and as a "plasticizer" (makes fixatives more flexible on the hair) in some hair setting products. Helps combing characteristics of hair products. Generally inert and non-toxic to skin. More water soluble than dimethicone. Silicones are organic/inorganic polymers consisting of long chains of alternating silicon and oxygen atoms. They are very stable and generally very water repellant, with low toxicity and low irritation potential. Also acts as emulsifiers in some systems.
Dipropylene Glycol (2-Methyl - 1, 3 Propanediol)	S	SOL, M	3-4	3-4	Solvent for fragrances and deodorants
Disodium Cocamido MIPA-Sulfosuccinate and Disodium Oleomido MIPA-Sulfosuccinate	V	CL	3	3	Very mild, non-drying cleansers/surfactants, with a mild conditioning effect. Helps reduce the irritation potential of other surfactants. Average foam and cleansing.
Disodium Cocoamphodiacetate	V	CL	3	3	A mild amphoteric cleanser often used in place of the stronger cleansing surfactants.

Ingredient Name/INCI Name (Other Names in Parentheses)	Source	Purpose	S	LCR	Notes
Disodium EDTA (Sodium salt of EDTA)	S	P, A	2	3	Often used as a chelating agent to remove trace heavy metals, such as iron, copper or lead, from a product. These heavy metals can be detrimental to the color, fragrance or other aesthetics of a formula and can destroy some vitamins. Usually used at concentrations below 0.2%. Very low toxicity. Some grades are approved for food use. Improves the activity of many preservatives.
Disodium Laureth Sulfosuccinate	V	CL	3	3	Mild, non-drying cleanser/surfactant, with a mild conditioning effect. Helps reduce the irritation potential of other surfactants. Average foam and cleansing.
Disodium Lauryl Sulfosuccinate	V	CL	3	3	Mild, non-drying cleanser/surfactant, with mild conditioning effect. Helps reduce the irritation potential of other surfactants. Average foam and cleansing.
Disodium Oleth-3 Sulfosuccinate	V	CL	3	2	A salt of substituted sulfosuccinic acid. Excellent foaming; low irritation. Leaves a "soft feel" on the skin.
(dl Panthenol) See "Panthenol"					
DMDM Hydantoin (1, 3-Dimethylol-5-5-dimethyl hydantoin)	S	P	4-5	4 RO 5 LV	May release formaldehyde as part of its preservative action. Preservative; developed as an odorless form of formaldehyde and designed to control its release.
Docosahexaenioc Acid (DHA)	A	A, M	1	3	An omega-3 fatty acid found mostly in cold water fish. Used internally for treatment of depression, schizophrenia and attention deficits.
(Docosanol) See "Behenyl Alcohol"					
(Dodecanol) See "Lauryl Alcohol"					
Dodecyl Laurate	V	E	3	3	Emulsifier and thickener

Ingredient Name/INCI Name (Other Names in Parentheses)	Source	Purpose	S	LCR	Notes
E					
Echinacea Extract (Purple cone flower, Echinacea Purpurea, Echinacea Angustifolia)	V	A	2	3	Anti-inflammatory; anti-bacterial and anti-viral. Believed to help boost immune system and heal wounds. Used to help heal acne and eczema. One active ingredient group is termed "echinacosides."
EDTA (See "Disodium EDTA")					
Eicosapentanoic Acid (EPA)	A, V	M, A	2	2	An Omega-3 polyunsaturated fatty acid usually from fish. Excellent moisturizer. Internally, believed to prevent heart attacks and cardiovascular disease, lower cholesterol, and improve cell membranes. It acts as an important agent in prostaglandin production, reducing inflammation and platelet aggregation.
(Elastin) See "Hydrolyzed Elastin"					
Elderberry Extract	V	A	2	2	Stimulates circulation; rich in vitamin C, flavonoids and tannins. Internally used to treat fever, muscle pain and flu symptoms.
Elder Flower Extract (Sambucus Nigra)	V	A	2	2	Used in treatment of various skin disorders; mild antiseptic; believed to soften skin and treat freckles and sunburn.
Ellagic Acid	V	O, A	2	2	An antioxidant from pomegranate (*Punica granatum*) and other fruits. Used as an anti-cancer and anti-viral agent.
Emulsifying Wax (Emulsifying Wax N.F., Polawax™)	V	E	2	2	Approved for use in cosmetics and pharmaceuticals. N.F. stands for "National Formulary," a pharmaceutical standard. Excellent all-purpose, safe, nonionic emulsifier. (Not a true wax)
(Epsom Salts) See "Magnesium Sulfate"					

Ingredient Name/INCI Name (Other Names in Parentheses)	Source	Purpose	S	LCR	Notes
Ergocalciferol	A, S	A	3	3 (At <0.1%)	A form of vitamin D. See "Cholecalciferol"
(Essential Fatty Acids) (See "Vitamin F")					Neither "essential fatty acids" or "vitamin F" is an approved label name.
Estrogen	S, A	A	3-5 (See page 20)	3-4	The female sex hormone, with anti-aging properties. Claimed to reverse thinning of hair, dry skin and mucous membranes, and to improve memory function.
(Ethanol) See "Ethyl Alcohol"					
Ethanolamine (MEA, Monoethanolamine)	S	pH	4	4	An amine used to neutralize acidic components or raise the pH. Also used as an intermediate to manufacture other ingredients.
Ethyl Acetate	S	SOL	4	5	Volatile solvent; often used in nail polishes
Ethyl Alcohol (Ethanol, Grain Alcohol)	V or S	SOL	4	4 LV 3 RO	Can dry, sting or irritate skin depending on concentration. OK for hair spray use, but avoid high concentrations in skin care LV products. Flammable in high concentrations. Maximum effectiveness for disinfection is about 70% concentration, and about 17% to act as an effective product preservative. Can remove the skin's protective lipids in high concentration. Ethyl alcohol is not the proper label name for denatured alcohol. (See "SD Alcohol 40," etc.)
Ethylene Glycol	S	M, SOL	5	4	Possible toxic effects if absorbed through the skin. (Do not confuse with Propylene Glycol)
Ethylene Glycol Stearate See "Glycol Stearate"					
Ethyl Ester of PVM/MA Copolymer	S	A	3	3	Polymer to help hold hair in place in hair fixative products, such as hair sprays and gels. (Ethyl ester of polycarboxylic resin)
Ethylhexyl Dimethyl PABA (Octyl Dimethyl PABA, Padimate O)	S	A	3	4	Sunscreen. LCR depends on concentration. The higher the SPF, the higher the likelihood of irritation. Less likely to cause a reaction than "PABA."

Ingredient Name/INCI Name (Other Names in Parentheses)	Source	Purpose	S	LCR	Notes
2-Ethylhexyl Methoxycinnamate (Octyl Methoxycinnamate)	S	A	3	4	Sunscreen. LCR depends on concentration. The higher the SPF, the higher the likelihood of irritation.
Ethylhexyl Palmitate (See "Octyl Palmitate")					
2-Ethylhexyl Salicylate (Octyl Salicylate)	S	A	3	4	Sunscreen. LCR depends on concentration. The higher the SPF, the higher the likelihood of irritation.
Ethyl Linoleate	V	M	2	2	Ester of linoleic acid, and internally used as a source of linoleic acid. Excellent "moisturizer" and skin nutrient. (See "Linoleic Acid")
Ethyl Panthenol	S	A, M	3	3	Ethyl ether derivative of panthenol. Believed to penetrate into the hair and moisturize better than panthenol. (See "Panthenol")
Ethyl Paraben	S	P	3	4	Usually used in 0.2% or less as a preservative.
Eucalyptus Oil (Eucalyptus Globulus)	V	F, A, P	3	4	Natural, pungent smelling oil. The odor will help you guess how much is present. Antiseptic. Also used as a fragrance or aromatherapeutic oil. Also used as a topical analgesic for pain relief.
Evening Primrose Oil (Oenothera Biennis)	V	M, A	2	3	Used as a source of essential fatty acids (EFA) - Linoleic and Linolenic (Omega-6) in particular. Highly recommend for skin. Helps repair/restore the intercellular moisture barrier of the skin. (Linoleic acid, 65-75%; gamma linolenic acid, 8-12%)
Eyebright Extract (Euphrasia Officinalis)	V	A	2	3	Anti-inflammatory; reduces redness and irritation. Has some astringent properties.

F

Ingredient Name/INCI Name (Other Names in Parentheses)	Source	Purpose	S	LCR	Notes
FD&C Yellow #5	S	C	4	4-5	Artificial color. FD&C means it is approved by the FDA for use in Foods, Drugs and Cosmetics.
FD&C Blue #1 (Brilliant Blue, Food Blue 2, C.I. 42090)	S	C	4	4	Artificial color. FD&C means it is approved by the FDA for use in Foods, Drugs and Cosmetics. (Triphenylmethane type.)
FD&C Green #3 (Fast green FCF, Food Green 3)	S	C	4	4	Artificial color. FD&C means it is approved by the FDA for use in Foods, Drugs and Cosmetics. (Triphenylmethane type.)
FD&C Red #40	S	C	4	4	Artificial color. FD&C means it is approved by the FDA for use in Foods, Drugs and Cosmetics.
Fennel Extract (Foeniculan Vulgare)	V	A, F	2	2	Anti-irritant, anti-inflammatory; moisturizer. Used for dry skin. The pure oil is used for fragrances, but may be more likely to elicit an allergic response than the aqueous extract.
Fibronectin	A	A	3	3	Protein used as a skin conditioner
Fir Oil	V	F	3	4	Fragrance and aromatherapeutic oil
Folic Acid	S	A	2	3	Member of the vitamin B group; a deficiency can cause megaloblastic anemia. Also needed for RNA/DNA synthesis. May help in skin repair.
Formaldehyde	S	P	5	5	Preservative; germicide; fungicide. "Formalin" is the name given to a solution of formaldehyde gas in water. Listed as "reasonably anticipated to be (a) human carcinogen" in the National Toxicology Program.
Fragrance	V or S or A	F	2-4	3-5	Usually a complex mixture of natural oils, synthetic oils or both. Sometimes as many as 200 different ingredients are used in a single fragrance.

Ingredient Name/INCI Name (Other Names in Parentheses)	Source	Purpose	S	LCR	Notes
Fructose (Fruit Sugar)	V	A	1	1	Sweetener; more sweet than sucrose
G					
(Gamma-Linolenic Acid) See "Linolenic Acid"					
(Gamma-Orizanol) or (Gamma-Oryzanol) See "Oryzanol"					
Garcinia Cambogia Extract (Indian Berry)	V	A	2	3	Used internally in weight reduction formulas. Active ingredient is hydroxycitric acid, HCA, which studies indicate blocks the production of fatty acids and cholesterol, making less fat available for storage. It also appears to reduce appetite by increasing the availability of glycogen in the liver.
Gardenia Oil (Gardenia Florida, Gardenia Tahitensis)	V	F	3	3 – 4 Depending on level	Fragrance or aromatherapeutic oil. Essential oil of gardenia flowers. As with most essential oils, the pure oil is much more likely to irritate than when it is used at a very low level as a fragrance.
Gelatin	A	A	3	3	Source of protein for hair and skin conditioning
Gentiana Lutea Extract	V	A	3	3	Anti-inflammatory
Geothermal Mixed Mineral Salts	M	A	2	2 RO or Bath use / 3 LV	Mineral salts from geothermal (hot springs), rich in special minerals believed to help heal various ailments. In Europe, soaking in these mineral baths is often doctor directed. (Called "taking the cure.") The mineral content varies depending on the source.
Geranium Oil (Geranium Maculatum)	V	F, A	3	3 – 4 Depending on level	Essential oil of geranium. Has astringent and antiseptic properties. Anti-bacterial.

Ingredient Name/INCI Name (Other Names in Parentheses)	Source	Purpose	S	LCR	Notes
Ginger Extract (Zingiber Officinale)	V (from leaves)	A	2	3	Mild tonic and skin soother. Counter irritant. Also used as a flavor. One active ingredient group is termed "gingerols." Has been used as a dandruff treatment. Internally used as a digestive aid and antinausea agent. (The seeds are toxic.)
Gingko Biloba Extract	V	A	1	2	In cosmetics, used as an antioxidant to help neutralize "free radicals" (believed to be a major cause of premature ageing). A recent study indicates that the flavanoid content enhances the fibroblast skin cells to produce more collagen and elastin. (See bibliography "10.") Vasodilator. Internally, widely accepted to affect regulation of blood flow to the brain, legs and other extremities. Used to treat cellulite and varicose veins. Actives are ginkgoflavonglucosides and triterpene lactones, usually 24% and 6% minimum respectively (24/6). (From the leaves.)
Ginseng Extract (Panax Ginseng - Chinese Panax Quinquifolium - American Eleutherococcus Senticosis - Siberian)	V	A	1	2	Extract used to normalize skin and make it less sensitive. Anti-irritant and hormonal regulator. Actives are ginsenosides (saponins). Internally, it is said to strengthen the body to help prevent and fight disease, increase stamina and counteract fatigue and stress.
Glucose	V	A	1	1	Grape or corn sugar
Glycereth - 7, 12, 26, etc.	V, S, A	M, E	2	3	Derived from Glycerin, used as a solubilizer, emulsifier, moisturizer and humectant.
Glycerin (Glycerine, Glycerol)	V, A, S	M	2	2	Made as a by-product of soap-making, or prepared synthetically. Good humectant but tends to be "sticky" on the skin if too high a level is used.
Glyceryl Cocoate	V	M	3	3	Emulsifier. Also used as an ointment base. (Ester of glycerin and coconut fatty acids)
Glyceryl Dilaurate	V	M, E	3	2	Nonionic emulsifier; emollient; solubilizer and de-tackifying aid. Provides a smooth, rich feel on the skin. Melts slightly below body temperature. Good emulsion stabilizer. (Diester of glycerin and lauric acid)

Ingredient Name/INCI Name (Other Names in Parentheses)	Source	Purpose	S	LCR	Notes
Glyceryl Linoleate	V	E, M	2	3	Emollient, emulsifier; source of linoleic acid. (Ester of glycerin and coconut linoleic acid)
Glyceryl Stearate (Glyceryl Monostearate)	V	E	2	2	Formed from reaction of glycerin and stearic acid; it is a mild, commonly used emulsifier that can also increase viscosity. (The material is actually a mixture of esters and un-reacted fatty acids, but predominantly glyceryl stearate). Some food-approved uses.
Glyceryl Stearate SE (Self-emulsifying)	V	E	2	3	Glyceryl stearate in which the unreacted stearic acid has been reacted with potassium hydroxide to produce a soap and thereby a self-emulsifying product.
Glyceryl Thioglycolate (Glyceryl Monothioglycolate)	S	A	4 – 5	5	Used in permanent waves to break the sulfide bonds in hair before the hair is reshaped. Known irritant. Main component of many "acid perms." See "Thioglycolic Acid"
Glycol Distearate	V	E, C	3	3	Thickener; emulsifier. Also used as an opacifier and "pearlizing" agent in shampoos.
Glycolic Acid	V, S	M, A, pH, Exf	3	3-5 (Avoid >10% and < pH 3.5)	An Alpha Hydroxy Acid, that in sufficient concentration, can exfoliate skin, producing a smoother skin surface. Concentration and pH is everything! Above about 7% or 8%, it is more likely to sting, burn or peel skin (at pHs below approximately 5). Component of sugar cane extract. Can increase UV induced photosensitivity of the skin. Can also increase skin tanning. Avoid high concentrations when you will be in the sun.
Glycol Stearate	V	E, C	3	3	Emulsifier. Also used as an opacifier and "pearlizing" agent in shampoos.
Glycyrrhizic Acid (Glycyrrhizinic Acid)	V	A	3	2	Main active ingredient of Licorice. Flavor, sweetener, anti-inflammatory. (See "Licorice Root Extract")
Goldenseal Extract (Hydrastis Canadensis)	V	A	3 (External)	3-4	Healing agent; mild antiseptic and antibiotic: astringent. Has been used on itchy skin, acne and inflammations. Do not ingest. Also used for eye and skin irritation treatment.

Ingredient Name/INCI Name (Other Names in Parentheses)	Source	Purpose	S	LCR	Notes
Gotu Kola Extract (Hydrocotyl, Centella Asiatica Extract)	V	A	2	3	Skin soother; healing agent; anti-inflammatory. Also used to treat burns, inflammation, acne, infection and cellulite. Claimed to stimulate collagen synthesis. Do not confuse with Kola Nut Extract. Actives are asiaticosides, triterpenes and madecassic acid. The triterpenes are reported to be capable of fixing alanine and proline into the structure of collagen, and thereby help promote healing of bedsores and skin disorders.
(Grain Alcohol) See "Ethyl Alcohol"					
Grapefruit Seed Extract (Citrus Grandis)	V	P, A	3	3	Preservative; bactericide; astringent. More than one type of extract is available. Low toxicity. While it is a mild, natural preservative, it is also a weak preservative, not effective in many products. Some extracts are used as anti-inflammatory and anti-acne agents. Some contain salicylic acid.
Grapeseed Extract (Vitis Vinifera)	V	O, A	1	3	Contains polyphenolic antioxidants, flavonoids and vitamin C. Anti-inflammatory. Contains proanthocyandins (antioxidants). Internally, claimed to have a positive effect against cholesterol, joint inflammation, ulcers and cataracts.
Grapeskin Extract (Vitis Vinifera)	V	C, O	1	2	Color; contains trans-resveratol, a phytoestrogen which is claimed to help prevent cancer (this is not proven). Also contains anthocyanidin antioxidants, which can support normal vision and improve capillary strength.
Green Tea Extract (Camellia Oleifera, Camellia Chenensis, Camellia Sinensis)	V	A, O	2	3	Excellent anti-oxidant. Contains polyphenols, natural anti-oxidants. Claimed to retard/prevent certain types of sun damage and cancer. Has astringent and anti-inflammatory properties. One of the primary actives is epigallocatechin-3-gallate. Claimed to help reinforce the skin's lipid barrier by stimulating ceramide production. Internally, also used as a digestive system protector. Some extracts contain the neurotransmitter GABA (gamma amino butric acid), known for its calming effects.

145

Ingredient Name/INCI Name (Other Names in Parentheses)	Source	Purpose	S	LCR	Notes
Guanine	A	C	3	3	A pearlizing agent from fish scales
Guarana Extract (Paullinia Cupana)	V	A	3	3	Source of caffeine; stimulant; tonic. Has astringent properties. Also used as a counter-irritant in some formulas.
Guar Gum (Cyanopsis Tetragonoloba)	V	T	2	2	Thickener and emulsion stabilizer. From the endosperm of the guar seed. High molecular weight polysaccharide, approved for food use.
Guar Hydroxypropyltrimonium Chloride (Quaternized Guar Gum)	V	A	3	3 RO 4 LV	Used as a conditioner, particularly in hair care product. Also used to help maximize deposition of silicones onto the hair, to aid in combing. (Cationic)
(Gum Arabic) See "Acacia"					
(Gum Benzoin) See "Benzoin Gum"					
Gum Karaya (Sterculia Urens)	V	T, S	2	3	From a tree in India, it is a complex polysaccharide. Acid resistant. Rarely used by itself because the developed viscosity tends to thin with age.
(Gum Tragacanth) See "Tragacanth Gum"					
H					
Hawthorne Extract (Crataegus Monogina)	V	A	3	3	Rich in OPC (oligomer proyanidin) antioxidants; internally used to increase coronary blood flow. Helps stabilize collagen.
Hectorite Clay	M	T, A	2	2	Natural suspending agent, gelling agent and thickener. Also used to draw out and absorb impurities when used in facial masks and acne products.

146

Ingredient Name/INCI Name (Other Names in Parentheses)	Source	Purpose	S	LCR	Notes
Henna Extract	V	C	3	3-4	Dried, powdered leaves used to color or tint hair. Better at bringing out the reddish highlights in most types of hair. There are several shades available, including a "neutral" henna which will not impart color to the hair, and is used as a hair conditioner. The active ingredient is "Lawsone," 2-hydroxy-1,4 naphthoquinone.
(Hemp Seed Oil) See "Cannabis Sativa Seed Oil"					The correct labeling name is "Cannabis Sativa Seed Oil."
Hexylene Glycol	S	SOL	3	3-4	Solvent and humectant
Honey	A	M	1	2-3	Emollient, humectant and bacteriostat. Some reports of pollen-allergic reaction. A recent study from Turkey suggests it may have anti-tumor properties in some uses.
Hops Extract	V	A	2	3	Antiseptic; tonic; astringent. Internally, it has a relaxing, calming effect. Used for oily skin, enlarged pores and bust care.
Horsechestnut Oil (Aesculus Hippocastanum)	V	A	2	3	Stimulating herb for treatment of scalp and skin conditions. Has some antibacterial properties. Claimed to increase blood circulation. The plant contains saponins. Some extracts contain proanthocyanidin antioxidants. Taken internally, it is claimed to help strengthen and repair capillaries and blood vessels, and to help varicose veins.
Horsetail Extract (Equisetum Arvense, Equisetum Hiemale)	V	A	2	3	A source of silicon (not "silicone") and also used as an astringent and antioxidant. Claimed to have healing properties by helping to stop bleeding, and used in treatment of varicose veins and circulatory problems. Primary active ingredient is escin, a mixture of saponins.

Ingredient Name/INCI Name (Other Names in Parentheses)	Source	Purpose	S	LCR	Notes
Hyaluronic Acid (Or its sodium salt "Sodium Hyaluronate")	V or A	M	1	1	Natural moisturizing component of human skin. Powerful moisturizer and "water magnet" that can bind 500 - 1000 times its own weight in water. As we age, the skin's hyaluronic acid content decreases. One of our most highly recommended ingredients. So safe it is used in eye surgery to keep the eye moist. A mucoploysaccharide of the glycosaminoglycan group (amino-sugar containing). (Most is derived from a fermentation process.)
Hydrocotyl (See "Gotu Kola Extract")					
Hydrogenated Vegetable Oils (See "Partially Hydrogenated Vegetable Oils")	V	M	2	3-4	Emollients; emulsifiers; cocoa butter replacement
Hydrogen Peroxide	M,S	Various	3-4	4	Bleaching agent; perm neutralizer; antibacterial agent. It is an oxidizing agent.
Hydrolysis (verb) - Hydrolyzed (adjective) (not an ingredient)					The process of breaking down larger molecules by means of acids, alkalines, heat and/or enzymes. For proteins this means reducing the molecular weight and the resulting smaller molecules are more water soluble.
Hydrolyzed Animal Protein	A	M, A	1	2-3	Can be from keratin or collagen sources
Hydrolyzed Elastin	A	M, A	1	2-3	Animal derived moisturizer for skin. Film-former. Elastin is found in the dermal tissues of animals, including humans. As we age, the elastin deteriorates somewhat. It is also negatively impacted by UV light.
Hydrolyzed Keratin Protein	H, A	M, A	1	2-3	Skin and hair conditioning protein prepared from actual hair by hydrolysis. The correct molecular weight (about 1,000 - 4,000) product is very substantive to hair and is used in a variety of hair care products.
Hydrolyzed Silk Protein	A	M, A	1	2-3	Moisturizer and conditioner for skin and hair care
Hydrolyzed Soy Protein	V	M, A	1	2-3	Moisturizer and conditioner for skin and hair care

Ingredient Name/INCI Name (Other Names in Parentheses)	Source	Purpose	S	LCR	Notes
Hydrolyzed Wheat Protein	V	M, A	1	2-3	Moisturizer and conditioner for skin and hair care. Comes in many forms, modified to increase substantivity.
Hydroquinone	S	A	5	5	Used as a skin bleach. Not permitted as an OTC drug in the U.S. if levels are above 2%. Can have serious side effects if applied over longer periods of time. Increases photosensitivity of skin. There are other ways of lightening the skin. (1) By chemically reacting with one or more of the intermediates that lead to melanin, or (2) by inactivating the key enzyme involved in melanin formation, tyrosinase.
Hydroxyethylcellulose and Hydroxyethyl Ethylcellulose	V	T	2	2	Cellulose derived stabilizers, suspending agents. Stable thickeners, used in a variety of water-based products - toothpastes, shampoos, etc. (Modified cellulose polymers.) (See "Cellulose Gum".)
Hydroxypropyl Methylcellulose (Carbohydrate Gum)	V	T	2	2	Derived from cellulose, and used as a thickener in a variety of personal care products. (See "Cellulose Gum")
Hydroxypropyltrimonium Hydrolyzed Wheat Protein	V	A	3	3	Conditioning agent for hair and skin. "Quaternized" wheat protein to increase substantivity.
I					
Imidazolidinyl Urea	S	P	3	3-4 RO 4-5 LV	Broad spectrum preservative, very water soluble. The molecule is closely related in structure to allantoin.
Iodopropynyl Butylcarbamate (IPBC)	S	P	5	4	Preservative; potent fungicide
Irish Moss Extract (Chondrus Crispus)	V	T, S	2	3	Natural carbohydrate mixture from seaweed, used to thicken, suspend and stabilize. (See "Carrageenan") Historically it has been used as a treatment for wounds. Also used as an emollient and to counteract dry skin and wrinkles.

149

Ingredient Name/INCI Name (Other Names in Parentheses)	Source	Purpose	S	LCR	Notes
Iron Oxides	M	C	2	4	Used as coloring pigments in make-up products. Available in a wide range of colors depending on the purity and amount of water present. Iron oxides can be produced synthetically. Super-heating is sometimes used to alter the pigment color ("burnt sienna" for example).
Isopropyl Alcohol (Isopropanol)	S, P	SOL	4	4-5 (At > 10%) 3-4 (At <10%)	Common solution in water is called "rubbing alcohol." Maximum effectiveness for disinfection is about 50% concentration. Can dry the skin and cause "cracking" in high concentrations. Do not ingest.
Isopropyl Palmitate and Isopropyl Myristate	V, S	M, E	3	3-4	Light, liquid esters used to reduce "tackiness" and provide a dry feel on the skin. Can be comedogenic in certain formulas and concentrations above approximately 5 - 7%. Odorless and colorless. Excellent "spreading" characteristics. Good formulation technique can eliminate likelihood of comedogenity.
Isopropyl Stearate	V, S, A	E, M	3	3	Mild emollient oil; emulsifier. Good "spreadability."
Isosteareth-10,20, etc.	V	E	3	3	Nonionic surfactants; emollients; solubilizing and emulsifying agents.
Isostearic Acid	V	E	3	4-5	Emulsifier with some emollient properties. A liquid isomer of stearic acid.
Isostearyl Linoleate	V	M	3	3	Moisturizing ester; also used to disperse color pigments.
Ivy Extract (Hedera Helix)	V	A	3	4	Used in the treatment of cellulite to stimulate circulation. Believed to have tonic properties.
J					
Jaboncillo Extract (Saponis Saponaria)	V	CL	3	2	Natural cleanser/foamer, rich in natural saponins. Also has some astringent properties.
Japan Wax	A	T	3	3	Not an ester; composed mainly of glyceryl tripalmitate with about 5% free fatty acids secreted by the insect, *Coccus ceriferus*.

Ingredient Name/INCI Name (Other Names in Parentheses)	Source	Purpose	S	LCR	Notes
Jasmine Oil (Jasminum Officinale)	V	F	3	4	Natural essential oil used for fragrance blends or aromatherapy
Jojoba Butter	V	M	2	3	Partially hydrogenated jojoba oil or jojoba oil altered under steam and pressure (Trans-isomerization). (Note: This product may vary in composition depending on the supplier.)
Jojoba Esters (Jojoba Creams)	V	M	2	3	This terminology is vague since jojoba naturally contains esters. It is believed to be partially hydrogenated jojoba oil or a selected higher melting point fraction of the jojoba oil esters, or a combination of the two.
Jojoba Oil (Buxus Chinensis, Simonsia Chinensis, Simmondsia Chinensis)	V	M	2	2	Unlike most vegetable oils, not a mixture of fatty acids. Resists oxidation (rancidity) better than vegetable oils. Resembles sperm whale oil in some respects. It is really liquid wax esters. Extracted from the seeds of a shrub found in the arid deserts of the American Southwest. Ideal lubricant and moisturizer. Some components have a structure similar to skin oil (sebum). Wide range of uses including dandruff prevention, massage oil, lubrication, healthy hair growth, shaving oil, body oil, make-up remover, etc. Non-comedogenic.
Jojoba Wax (Jojoba Beads, Hydrogenated Jojoba Oil)	V	Exf	2	3	The waxy beads are used as a very light, mild exfoliant, generally used where very little exfoliation is desired. Avoid the eye area. Also used as a wax in lipsticks, lip balms, and as an occlusive moisturizer in other products.
Juniper Extract (Juniperus Communis, Juniperus Oxycedrus)	V	A, F	3	3-4 Depending on concentration	Used as a flavor or fragrance. Has astringent properties; anti-inflammatory. Used for an oily skin treatment. The berries are an antiseptic and antibiotic. The oil is used in the preparation of gin.

K

(K Vitamin) See "Phytonadione"					

Ingredient Name/INCI Name (Other Names in Parentheses)	Source	Purpose	S	LCR	Notes
Kaolin (China Clay; Bolus Alba)	M	A, T	2	2	Silicate clay used as an absorbant in masks, face powder and occasionally as a thickener. Helps remove the shine produced by talc. Able to absorb large amounts of oil or moisture. There are many types and grades of kaolin.
Karaya Gum (Sterculia Urens)					(See "Gum Karaya")
Kava-Kava Extract (Piper Methysticum)	V	A	3	3	Internally, it has a sedative effect. Can induce restful sleep and treat fatigue and anxiety. Herbal muscle relaxant. Has antiseptic properties applied topically. Active ingredients are kava pyrones.
Kelp or Kelp Extract (Laminaria Digitata, Macrocystis Pyrifera)	V	A, M	1	2	Stimulates circulation; remineralizer; moisturizer; used in anti-cellulite treatments. Rich in iodine. An important part of the diet in Japan.
(Keratin) See "Hydrolyzed Keratin Protein"	A		1	2	Non-hydrolyzed keratin is rarely used in cosmetics. Keratin is an insoluble protein which makes up the greater part of hair and wool. Like other proteins, it is composed of amino acids.
Keratin Amino Acids	H, A	A, M	2	3	Used as a hair or skin conditioner and moisturizer. Keratin is a protein found in hair, wool, nails and skin. (See "Hydrolyzed Keratin")
Kiwi Extract (Actinidia Chinensis)	V	A	2	3	Tonic; skin and hair conditioner
Kiwi Fruit Seed Oil (Actinidia Chinensis)	V	M	2	3	High in linoleic acid (15-24%) and alpha linoleic acid (45-70%); omega-3 fatty acid source.
Kojic Acid	V, S	A	3	4	Bleaching agent; skin whitening ingredient. Generally unstable in an aqueous base. Commonly prepared by carbohydrate fermentation.
Kola Nut Extract (Cola Nitida, Cola Acuminata)	V	A	1	2	Anti-irritant, used to reduce the likelihood of a formula to irritate the skin. Source of caffeine (about 3 - 10%).

Ingredient Name/INCI Name (Other Names in Parentheses)	Source	Purpose	S	LCR	Notes
Kukui Oil or Kukui Nut Oil (Aleurites Moluccana)	V	M	2	3	Oil from a Hawaiian nut with very good emollient and moisturizing properties. Rich in essential fatty acids, linoleic acid (35-45%) and alpha linolenic acid (25-35%).
L					
Lactamide MEA	V, S	M	3	3	Moisturizer and humectant. Derived from lactic acid. Nonionic antistatic agent and conditioner.
Lactic Acid (L (+) - lactic acid)	V	A, pH, M	2	3 or 4 (at higher levels)	Along with glycolic acid, one of the two most common alpha hydroxy acids. Occurs in sour milk, molasses and many fruits, and in the human body. Also prepared commercially via fermentation. Also used at lower levels in products as a humectant and pH adjuster. In very high concentrations, it can be irritating to skin (>about 8.0%). Additionally, it has humectant and antimicrobial properties D (-) - lactic acid is not recommended, as it is more irritating.
Lactose (Milk Sugar)	A, S	A	1	2	Sweetener; humectant
Laminaria (See "Kelp")					
Laneth-5, 10, 15, 20 etc.	A	M, E	3	4	Nonionic ethoxylated lanolin. Gelling agents, emollients and solubilizers.
Lanolin	A	M	3	4-5	Chemically, closest of all natural raw materials to human sebum. From sheep's wool (the fat-like secretion of the sheep's sebaceous glands). Chemically, it is a wax rather than a fat or oil, and a complex mixture of esters of various alcohols. Occlusive type moisturizer and emulsifier. Can cause a skin reaction in some people. Possible common allergen. Different suppliers can produce differing purities of lanolin, resulting in varying degrees of irritation potential.

Ingredient Name/INCI Name (Other Names in Parentheses)	Source	Purpose	S	LCR	Notes
Lanolin Alcohol	A	M	3	4	Complex fatty alcohol, derived from wool lanolin, has some humectant properties and is a source of cholesterol in cosmetic products. Normally used at 0.5 - 3.0 % in formulas.
Lanolin Oil	A	M, SOL	3	4	The "lighter" (lower melting point) parts of lanolin. Occlusive type moisturizer.
Lauramide DEA	V	T, CL	3-4	4	Thickener, cleanser, solubilizer and/or foam booster, commonly used in shampoos and bath gels. (An "Alkanolamide") (See "Cocamide DEA") Made from a lauric acid group and DEA (diethanolamine).
Lauramide MEA and Lauramide MIPA	V	T, CL	3	3	Thickener, cleanser, solubilizer and/or foam booster, commonly used in shampoos and bath gels. (An "Alkanolamide") Made from a lauric acid group and MEA (monoethanolamine), or MIPA (monoisopropanolamine).
Lauramidopropyl Betaine	V	CL	3	3	Mild amphoteric cleansing surfactant; foam enhancer and thickener
Lauramidopropyl Dimethylamine	V	A	3	3-4	Cationic emulsifier with enhanced substantivity to skin and hair. Lower irritation than normal quaternary conditioners. Anti-static agent.
Laureth - 1, 4, 9, 12, etc.	V	E	3	3	Nonionic emulsifiers, made from lauryl fatty alcohol. There is some belief that the lower the number, the greater the likelihood of irritation.
Lauric Acid (Dodecanoic Acid)	V	M	3	3-4	Natural fatty acid used as an emulsifier, wetting agent and intermediate to produce a variety of cosmetic raw materials. Primarily derived from coconut or palm kernel oils.
Laurydimonium Hydroxypropyl Hydrolyzed Collagen	A	A	3	4	Collagen protein which has been transformed into a "Quat" compound for improved conditioning, substantivity and antistatic electricity effect.
Lauryl Alcohol (Dodecanol)	V	T, E	3	3	Natural fatty alcohol from lauric acid. Used as an emulsifier, emollient and in the manufacture of many cosmetic raw materials.
Lauryl Betaine	V	CL	3	3	Mild cleansing amphoteric surfactant, foam enhancer and thickener

154

Ingredient Name/INCI Name (Other Names in Parentheses)	Source	Purpose	S	LCR	Notes
Lauryl Lactate	V	M	3	3	Liquid alpha hydroxy acid ester, used as an emollient
Lavender Extract (or Oil) (Lavandula Angustifolia)	V	F, A	3	3	Used as a fragrance essential oil and in aromatherapy. Antiseptic. Used in acne treatments and for irritated skin. Used as a hair and scalp tonic and to help prevent loss of hair.
Lead Acetate	M	A	5	5	Avoid. Used in hair darkeners to cover gray. Lead has a high toxicity. Avoid using near eyes or open wounds or sores. Listed as "Reasonably anticipated to be (a) human carcinogen" in the National Toxicology Program.
Lecithin (Phosphatidyl Choline)	V	M, E	2	3	From soybeans (can be prepared from eggs). A phospholipid present in all living cells. Commonly used as an emulsifier, but excellent as a moisturizer. Employed in the creation of liposomes. Rich in inositol.
Lemon Extract (Citrus Medica Limonum or Citrus Limonum)	V	F, A	2	3-4 5 (pure oil)	Astringent; antiseptic. Used to help oily skin or enlarged pores. The pure oil is more likely to irritate than the low level used in fragrances.
Lemongrass Extract (or Oil) (Cymbopogon Schoenanthus or Cymbopogon Citratus)	V	F, A	2	2	Used as an essential fragrance oil or in aromatherapy. Also used as insect repellant due to its citronella content.
Lichen Plant Extract (Usnea Barbata)	V	P	2	3-4	Used as an antibacterial in deodorants and other products.
Licorice Root Extract (Glycyrrhiza Glabra)	V	A	3	2-3	Skin soother; anti-irritant; anti-inflammatory. Source of glycyrrhizen, a sapon-like glycoside and sweetening agent. Claimed to suppress secretion of the scalp's sebum. Source of phytoestrogens also, depending on the particular extract. (Note: Many common so-called licorice flavors are really anise oil - not licorice.)
Lime Oil (Citrus Aurantifolia, Citrus Medica, Citrus Acris)	V	F	2	3	Used in flavors and fragrances. Has astringent properties. The juice is also used in the manufacture of citric acid.

Ingredient Name/INCI Name (Other Names in Parentheses)	Source	Purpose	S	LCR	Notes
Linoleic Acid	V	M	1	2	An essential fatty acid and constituent of many vegetable oils. Excellent for skin health. (An omega-6 unsaturated fatty acid.)
Linolenic Acid (and Gamma-Linolenic Acid, GLA)	V	A, M	2	3	Anti-inflammatory; skin nourisher; helps maintain skin flexibility. Maintains epidermal water barrier. Can help prevent excema. A polyunsaturated essential fatty acid, which must be provided by diet. Gamma-Linolenic Acid is an omega-6 fatty acid. Found in borage, black current and evening primrose oils. GLA is a precursor for PEG-1 prostaglandins, which have anti-inflammatory, skin health and vasodilatory properties. Alpha Linolenic Acid is an omega-3 fatty acid.
Lion's Mane Extract or Lion's Mane Mushroom Extract (Hericium Erinaceus, Monkey's Head)	V	A	1	2	The mushroom contains anti-cancer, and antibiotic compounds. Rich in immune-boosting polysaccharides. The extracts may vary greatly in active content.
(a-Lipoic Acid) See "a-Lipoic Acid" under "A"					
Lithospermun Extract [Lithospermum Officinale, Lithospermum Erythrorhizon, Zi Cao (China)]	V	A	3	2-3	UV absorber, skin protectant. There are several types of extracts from the plant (from China and Japan). Depending on what is extracted, it may be used as an anti-inflammatory, burn or excema treatment or for other skin disorders. Some extracts can be used as a natural color, which varies depending on the pH. The root contains naphthazarine (color) pigments which yield alkannin and shikonin. Alkannin is a color pigment (AKA, anchusin).
Live Yeast Cell Extract	V	A, M	2	3	Anti-irritant; healing agent

Ingredient Name/INCI Name (Other Names in Parentheses)	Source	Purpose	S	LCR	Notes
Locust Bean Gum (Ceratonia Siliqua, Carob Bean Gum)	V	T, S	2	2	Anti-irritant; thickener. High molecular weight polysaccharide. Interacts with kappa carrageenan to increase gel strength and elasticity. From the endosperm of the carob or locust seed. Approved for food use. Thickener; film-former; skin protectant. Produces a high viscosity.
(L-Selenomethionine) (See "Selenomethionine")					
Luffa (or Loofa) (Luffa Cylindrica)	V	Exf	1	2	The ground-up material is used as an exfoliant in body scrubs. It is from the dried fruit of the natural sponge - *luffa cylindrica*. Do not use the small particles near the eye area.
Lutein	V	O	1	2	A protective carotenoid antioxidant used to protect against UV damage. Internally, used to fight age-related macular degeneration.
Lycopene	V	O	1	2	Antioxidant found in many fruits. Can help reduce sun damage to the skin. Occurs mainly as the red pigment in tomatoes. Member of the carotenoid family (like beta-carotene). Internally used as an anti-cancer agent. Not naturally produced in the human body - must be supplemented. Also claimed to help reduce cholesterol when taken internally.
M					
Macadamia Nut Oil	V	M	2	3	Provides good penetration of the top skin layers; emollient.
Magnesium Aluminum Silicate	M	T, S	2	2	Natural mineral (smectite clay) used as a suspending and thickening agent in water based products. Also helps stabilize emulsions. Some grades are approved for use in pharmaceuticals.
Magnesium Ascorbyl PCA	V, S	A, O	2	3	More stable form of ascorbic acid. Releases ascorbic acid in the skin.

Ingredient Name/INCI Name (Other Names in Parentheses)	Source	Purpose	S	LCR	Notes
Magnesium Ascorbyl Phosphate (MAP)	M, V, S	A, O	2	3	More stable form of ascorbic acid. Very effective at whitening skin by means of inhibiting melanin formation. Made from ascorbic acid. Antioxidant. Releases ascorbic acid in the skin by the action of natural phosphatase enzymes.
Magnesium Carbonate	M	A	2	3	Used in powders as an absorbant (better than calcium carbonate). Tends to dry the skin. Helps create a "fluffiness" in powder blends.
Magnesium Sulfate (Epsom Salts)	M	A	3	2-4	Source of Magnesium Common in bath salts to soothe aches and pains
Maitake Extract or Maitake Mushroom Extract (Grifola Frondosa. Chinese - Wu Ron)	V	A	1	2	Used for its immune-enhancing effects. High beta-glucan content.
Marigold Extract See "Calendula Extract"					
(Marshmallow Root) See "Althea Extract"					
Mate Extract (Ilex Paraguariensis)	V	A	3	3	Source of caffeine: stimulant; circulation enhancer.
Matracaria Extract (See "Chamomile Extract")					
MEA (Abbreviation for Monoethanolamine, or Monoethanolamide - when used as a suffix)	S	A:, pH	3-4	3-4	Used to neutralize acidic compounds. When you see MEA as a suffix or prefix, it means a new molecule has been formed. There may or may not be any "free" MEA remaining in the new ingredient, depending on the process.

Ingredient Name/INCI Name (Other Names in Parentheses)	Source	Purpose	S	LCR	Notes
Meadowfoam Seed Oil (Limnanthes Alba)	V	A	3	3	Skin and hair conditioner; emollient
MEA – Thioglycolate	S	A	5	5	Permanent wave active ingredient See "Thioglycolic Acid."
Menthol	V, S	A, F	3	3-5	A naturally occurring constituent of peppermint oil. Used for its cooling effect, counter-irritant and antiseptic properties. Concentration about 1.0% or above can irritate skin or mucus membranes. Skin reaction depends on the level to a large degree.
Methenamine (Hexamine)	S	pH, P	5	5	Antiseptic; deodorant; preservative. Formaldehyde is released during hydrolysis.
Methyl Cellulose	V	T, S	2	2	Cellulose derived thickener. Somewhat incompatible with glycerin.
Methyl Gluceth-20 and Methyl Gluceth-10	V, S	E, M	2	2	Derived from glucose; humectants; emulsifiers. Also used as solubilizers. Ethoxylate stearate esters of naturally derived methyl glucose. Ethylene oxide free.
Methyl Glucose Sequistearate	V, S	E	2	2	Glucose derived nonionic emulsifier; a stearate ester of corn or palm derived methyl glucose.
Methyl Glucose Trioleate	V,S	E, T	3	3	Glucose derived emulsifier, used primarily as a thickener in cleansers and shampoos.
Methylparaben	S	P	3-4	3-4	Preservative, usually used in concentrations at 0.2% or less. Particularly effective against fungus and mold. Parabens can be inactivated by nonionic emulsifiers. Food approved for some uses. The most water soluble of the parabens. As with all preservatives, in general our opinion is, the lower the level, the less likelihood of irritation. Unlike many preservatives, parabens are not formaldehyde donors.
Methyl Salicylate (Oil of Wintergreen)	V, S	A, F	4-5	4-5	Used as a flavoring, counter-irritant, and for its cooling effect. Can be toxic if taken internally.

Ingredient Name/INCI Name (Other Names in Parentheses)	Source	Purpose	S	LCR	Notes
Methylsilanol Mannuronate	S, M, V	A	2	2-3	Anti-irritant; skin protectant; exceptional moisturizer. Source of silicon. Also has antioxidant and anti-inflammatory properties. Used in products for sensitive and acne skin. Also used in some anti-cellulite products.
Mexican Yam Extract (See "Wild Yam Extract")					
Mica	M	C	3	3	Used to create a "pearly" look to a liquid product. It can also improve skin feel and skin adhesion in powder products. Also used as a "filler" and oil-absorbing aid.
Microcrystalline Wax (Petroleum Wax)	P	E, T	4-5	4	A paraffin wax. Used to help thicken a variety of products. There are several grades available, varying in the mixture of hydrocarbons.
Milk-Thistle Extract (Silybum Marianum)	V	A	2-3	2-3	Anti-oxidant. Source of silymarin, an antioxidant and flavonoid complex, used to treat liver problems and organ toxicity. See "Silymarin"
Mineral Oil (Paraffin Oil)	P	M	3-5	4	Hydrocarbon. Petroleum derived lubricant and emollient oil. More occlusive than fruit and vegetable oils. Use started early in the twentieth century as a replacement for the less stable vegetable oils. Widely used because it is stable, easily available and inexpensive. (It is the mixture of the high boiling distillates from crude oil.) Mineral oils are listed as known carcinogens in the "National Toxicology Program." It may be that it is the "contaminant" hydrocarbons that are the carcinogens, not the oil itself.
Mink Oil	A	M	3	3	Animal derived emollient oil
Mistletoe Extract (Viscum Album)	V	A	3	3	Vasodilator
Montan Wax	M, V	T	3	3-4	Derived from lignite, a partially mineralized vegetable product, related to bituminous coal.

Ingredient Name/INCI Name (Other Names in Parentheses)	Source	Purpose	S	LCR	Notes
Montmorillonite Clay	M	T	2	2	A natural clay used for thickening or suspending other ingredients, or stabilizing a formula.
Myristyl Alcohol	V	E	2	3	Fatty alcohol from myristic acid
Myristyl Lactate	V	E, M	3	3	Emollient; emulsifier
Myristyl Myristate	V	E, M	3	3	A "dry feeling" emollient, that can increase viscosity. Melts at body temperatures.
Myrrh Oil (Commiphora Myrrha or Commiphora Molmol)	V	A, F	3	3	Essential oil for fragrances or aromatherapy. Has antiseptic and astringent properties. Used for treating wounds. A mixture of gum, resin and essential volatile oils.
N					
Neroli Oil	V	F	3	3-5 Depending on concentration	Essential oil of orange flower. The pure oil can be irritating to skin.
Nettle Extract (Urtica Dioica)	V	A	2	3	The extract is used as a hair conditioner and hair rinse to help restore natural color. Said to stimulate hair growth when applied to the scalp. It has also been used as an external treatment for rheumatic pains, as a topical analgesic.
Neutral Henna Extract (Lawsonia Inermis)	V	A, C	3	4	See "Henna Extract"
Niacin (Nicotinic Acid)	V, S	A	2	3	Vitamin B_3 – minute amounts occur in all living cells. Necessary for proper skin health. Used in cellulite and scalp treatments to increase circulation (rubefacient). Dilates blood vessels if taken internally. A deficiency can lead to dermatitis. Necessary for regeneration of the antioxidant - glutathione.
Niacinamide (Nicotinamide)	V, S	A	2	3	Pro-vitamin B_3. Occurs in plants and animals. Used in cellulite and scalp treatments to increase circulation.

Ingredient Name/INCI Name (Other Names in Parentheses)	Source	Purpose	S	LCR	Notes
Nitrocellulose	V	A	4	4-5	The basis of many nail polishes - the film forming resin.
Nonoxynol-1, 2, 4, etc.	S, P	E	3	3-4	The nonoxynol series has a variety of uses - emulsifiers, solubilizers and surfactants.
Nucleic Acids	A, S, H	A	2	3	A large class of acids, the two most studied are ribonucleic acid (RNA) and deoxyribonucleic acid (DNA). (See RNA/DNA)
Nylon-12	S	A	2	2	Absorbant powder; excellent in oily skin products. Essentially inert.
O					
Oak Bark Extract (Quercus Robur, Quercus Marliandica)	V	A	2	3	Astringent. Also a source of proanthocyanidin anti-oxidants.
Oat Bran Extract (Avena Sativa)	V	A	1	2	For treatment of dry skin: skin soother.
Oat Flour (Avena Sativa)	V	A	1	2	Skin soother; anti-irritant. Treatment for dry skin. Plant source of albumin and gluten. Skin protectant in some OTC drug products.
Octacosanol	V	A	1	2	Nutrient to increase stamina and athletic performance. Wheat germ oil is a good source. Unable to find topical uses.
(Octadecanol) See "Stearyl Alcohol"					
Octadecyl Stearate	V	E	3	3	Emulsifier and thickener
Octocrylene	S, P	A	3	4	Sunscreen
Octyl Dimethyl PABA (See "Ethylhexyl Dimethyl PABA")					

Ingredient Name/INCI Name (Other Names in Parentheses)	Source	Purpose	S	LCR	Notes
Octyldocenanol (1-dodecanol, 2-octyl)	V	E, M	2	3-4	Liquid fatty alcohol; emollient; color pigment dispersant; solubilizer.
Octyldodecyl Erucate	V	M	3	3	Liquid, dry feeling emollient ester
Octyl Isononanoate	S	A, M	2	2	Emollient; solvent, wetting agent
(Octyl Methoxycinnamate) See "2-Ethylhexyl Methoxycinnamate"					
Octyl Octanoate	V, S	M	3	3	Emollient
Octyl Palmitate (2-Ethylhexyl Palmitate)	V	E, M	2	3	Derived from palmitic acid, it is a light, non-greasy liquid used to reduce tackiness, help emulsify and produce a smooth feel on the skin. Can increase "shine" in some formulas.
Octyl Salicylate See "2-Ethylhexyl Salicylate"					
Octoxynol-1, 3, 5, etc.	S, P	E	3-4	3-4	Emulsifiers; solubilizers; dispersants; surfactants. (Ethoxylated alkyl phenols)
Oleamide DEA	V	E, CL, T	4	3-4	Emulsifier; thickener; foam booster; like most DEA neutralized ingredients, it may contain free DEA (diethanolamine), depending on the supplier and process.
Oleic Acid	V, A	E	3	3-5	Natural liquid, unsaturated fatty acid. Can be irritating or comedogenic in higher concentrations.
Oleth-2	S	E	3	4	A solubilizer, commonly used in bath oils to help disperse the oils in water.
Oleth - 3, 5, 10, 20, etc.	V	M, E	3	3-4	Nonionic emulsifiers and solubilizers. They become more water soluble and, in general, less likely to cause irritation as the number increases. Derived from oleyl alcohol.

Ingredient Name/INCI Name (Other Names in Parentheses)	Source	Purpose	S	LCR	Notes
Oleth - 3 Phosphate	V	E	3	3-4	Oil in water emulsifier; particularly used for clear, micro-emulsion gels. A phosphate ester. The higher the number, the less likely the potential for irritation.
Oleth - 10, 20, etc. Phosphate	V	E	3	3-4	Oil in water emulsifiers; particularly used for clear, micro-emulsion gels. They are phosphate esters. The higher the number, the less likely the potential for irritation.
Oleyl Alcohol	V, A	E, M	3	4	A liquid emulsifier and emollient. Also used as a color pigment suspending agent in lipsticks. Low viscosity, non-tacky oil. Used as a coupling agent and solvent in some formulas.
Oleyl Betaine	V, A	CL	3	3	Mild amphoteric surfactant
Olive Oil (Olea Europaea)	V	M	1	3	Believed to have many healing and protective properties. Used as an emollient and lubricant in skin and hair care formulas. Used as a primary oil in the manufacture of soap and a few surfactants. Moderate source of omega-6 fatty acids.
Olive Oil Glutinate	V	CL, E	3	2-3	Made from a wheat protein amine group and olive oil.
Orange Oil (Citrus Aurantium Dulcis)	V	F	3	3-5 Depending on concentration	Used as a flavor or fragrance oil. Has astringent properties.
Orange Peel Extract (Citrus Aurantium Dulcis)	V	F, A	2	3-4	Astringent; anti-cellulite ingredient; the oil portion is commonly used as a fragrance.
Oryzanol (Gamma Oryzanol)	V	A	2	3	Antioxidant and sunscreen from rice hulls and/or rice bran oil. Not approved for use as a protective sunscreen in the U.S.
(Oxybenzone) See "Benzophenone-3"					

Ingredient Name/INCI Name (Other Names in Parentheses)	Source	Purpose	S	LCR	Notes
Ozokerite (Mineral Wax, Ceresin)	P	T	4	3-4	Used to help raise the melting point in stick type products and increase the toughness of the stick. A hydrocarbon wax; some types contain mineral oil. True ozokerite is found only in specific petroleum deposits and is rarely available. What is called "ozokerite" today is usually a blend of petroleum waxes, that attempts to duplicate its features. Many grades are available.
P					
PABA (Para-Aminobenzoic Acid, p-Aminobenzoic Acid, Amino Benzoic Acid)	V, S	A	3	4-5 (At >1%) 3-4 (At <1%)	Commonly found in many foods and produced in the human body. Part of the folic acid molecule and member of the vitamin B complex. Sunscreen. Believed to be moderately likely to cause a skin reaction (at the higher levels commonly found in sunscreens), and has poor solubility except in alcohol. For these reasons, it is rarely used, except at very low levels (less than about 0.5%), to protect the color in certain products. Reported to be a sensitizer at sunscreen use levels (about 5%). More typically used today are its milder esters like octyl dimethyl PABA. Not so likely to irritate in concentrations less than about 0.5%, when used as a UV protector to protect the product itself.
(Palma Christi Oil) See "Castor Oil"					
Palmitoyl Pentapeptide - 3	V, S	M, A	3	2-3	Prepared by reaction of palmitic acid with amino acid groups.
Palmkernelamide DEA	V	T, CL	3	3	Used as a foam booster, cleanser and thickener in shampoos and bath gels. (Ethanolamides of fatty acids derived from palm kernel oil)
Pantethine	S	M, A	2-3	2-3	Hair conditioner; moisturizer. Used to improve the strength of hair, by binding free disulfide links in the hair.

Ingredient Name/INCI Name (Other Names in Parentheses)	Source	Purpose	S	LCR	Notes
Panthenol	V, S	A	2	2	Provitamin B-5. Used as a hair and skin conditioner. Has moisturizing and humectant qualities. There is data supporting the claim that it will also increase the size of each hair shaft when used in sufficient concentration (about 2% - 5%). Believed to convert in the hair to pantothenic acid. Does not build up on the hair. Helps protect hair from heat damage.
Dexpanthenol-natural dl-Panthenol-synthetic (only 50% active compared to Dexpanthenol)					Helps relieve minor burns, sunburn and reddened skin. A much more stable form of pantothenic acid. Helps accelerate wound healing. Reduces nail breakage and increases flexibility.
Pantothenic Acid	V, S	A	2	2	Essential body nutrient. Panthenol is converted by the body into pantothenic acid. An internal deficiency can cause graying of the hair. Used in the treatment of scalp diseases and wound healing. (See "Panthenol")
Papain (From "Carica Papaya")	V	A, Exf	2	3	Papaya enzyme is used as a mild exfoliant in light skin peels.
Papaya Enzyme (From "Carica Papaya")					See "Papain"
Paper Mulberry Extract (Broussonetia Kazinoki Seibold or B. Papyrifera)	V	A	3	3	The root bark extract of this tree contains tyrosinase inhibitors. Regular use can lighten skin tone by preventing normal melanin formation.
Paraffin (Paraffin Wax)	P	T, S	4-5	3-4	Stabilizer and thickener. Composed of straight-chain hydrocarbons.
(Paraffin Oil) See "Mineral Oil"					

Ingredient Name/INCI Name (Other Names in Parentheses)	Source	Purpose	S	LCR	Notes
Partially Hydrogenated Vegetable Oils (Soybean, Safflower, etc.)	V	M	2	3-4	In order to make vegetable oils less prone to rancidity, more "shelf stable" or to raise their melting point, the natural oils are treated with hydrogen to partially alter the molecular structure. (This process can destroy some vitamins, such as A and D.)
Passionflower Oil	V	M	2	3	Contains a high level of Linoleic Acid.
PCA (See "Sodium PCA")					
PEG					Abbreviation for "Polyethylene Glycol." As a prefix, it usually refers to a polymer of ethylene oxide.
PEG-4, 75, PEG-100, etc.	S	T, E	4	3-4	Used for a variety of purposes - thickening, lubricity, emulsifying, suspending, humectant action and as solvents. Some are approved for pharmaceutical use.
PEG-8 Beeswax	A, S	T, M	3	3	Sometimes used to increase the melting point of lipsticks.
PEG-30, 35, etc., Castor Oil	V	E, SOL	3	3	Emulsifiers; solubilizers
PEG-2 Cocoamide	V	CL, E, T	3	3	A primary amide made from coconut oil. This molecule substantially reduces the risk of nitrosamine formation.
PEG-4, 5, 6, etc., Dilaurate	V, S	E	3	3-4	Emulsifiers; solubilizers
PEG-150 Distearate (PEG-4000 Diisostearate)	V or A	E	3	3	Emulsifier, thickener (made from stearic acid). Used primarily in surfactant based cleansers to thicken the formula. (See "PEG-8 Stearate")
PEG-7 Glyceryl Cocoate	V	E, CL	3	3-4	Emulsifier and surfactant
PEG-30, 60, 75, etc. Lanolin	A	M, E	3	3-4	Conditioners; emulsifiers; emollients. Can be used to increase viscosity and stabilize foam.

Ingredient Name/INCI Name (Other Names in Parentheses)	Source	Purpose	S	LCR	Notes
PEG-2 Laurate	V	E	3	3-4	An emulsifier. A reaction product of lauric fatty acid and a 2-molar PEG polymer. (See "PEG")
PEG-120 Methyl Glucose Dioleate and PEG-120 Methyl Glucose Trioleate	V	CL, T	3	2	Corn-derived surfactant cleansers. Sometimes blended with other more "harsh" surfactants to increase the mildness of the final product. Reduces irritation potential of formulas. Also used to thicken some formulas.
PEG-10 Soya Sterol	V	M, E, A	3	3	Naturally derived emulsifier and emollient. The reaction product of soya sterol and a PEG polymer. (See "Soya Sterol")
PEG-8 Stearate	V or A	E, T	3	3	Used as an emulsifier and thickener. The reaction product of stearic acid and a PEG polymer. (See "PEG")
PEG-20, 100, etc. Stearate	V or A	E	3	3	Commonly used nonionic emulsifiers for creams and lotions, made from stearic acid. Can also be used to increase viscosity in creams and lotions. (See "PEG-8 Stearate")
Pennyroyal Oil (Mentha Pulegium)	V	A, F	4	4-5	Used as a deodorant, insect repellant and fragrance oil. Used in flea and mosquito repellants. (The pure oil itself is quite toxic - avoid.)
Pentaerythrityl Tetraisostearate (PTIS)	S	S, T, E, M	3	3-4	Used to thicken, suspend pigments and solubilize suncreens.
Peppermint Oil (Mentha Piperita)	V, S	F, A	3	3 - RO 4-5 LV, Depending on concentration	Used for cooling and antiseptic properties in many products. (High menthol content, 30 - 70%.) Also used as a flavor and fragrance. Internally, it is a digestive aid and breath freshener.
Perfluorononyl Dimethicone	M	A	3	3	Fluorine modified silicone, to increase substantivity and produce a lighter, more satiny skin feel.

Ingredient Name/INCI Name (Other Names in Parentheses)	Source	Purpose	S	LCR	Notes
Petrolatum (Petroleum Jelly)	P	M	3-4	4	Inexpensive hydrocarbon from petroleum. Occlusive moisturizer. Effective at preventing environmental damage to skin in harsh climates. Greasiness is a primary drawback. Many of the problems and questions about petroleum-derived hydrocarbons are believed to relate to impurities within them. (See "Mineral Oil" - both are from petroleum)
Phenoxyethanol (Rose Ether)	S, V	P	3	3	Preservative; topical antiseptic. One of the milder preservatives for cosmetics. Low toxicity – even when ingested.
Phospholipid Liposomes	V	A	2	2	See "Liposomes" in "terms" section of this book. Phospholipids are normally derived from lecithin. The principal phospholipid in lecithin is phosphatidylcholine. Other sources are egg yolks and soy (glycine max). (See "Lecithin")
Phytantriol	S	M	2	3	Hair and skin moisturizer
Phytonadione (Vitamin K)	S	A	3	3-5 Depending on concentration and formula	Used to stimulate circulation in foot and leg products. Do not use on the face in high concentrations, as it may redden skin. In low concentrations, it can be used as a treatment for dark circles under the eyes. Has anti-bacterial activity. Internally, it promotes normal growth and development and is necessary for blood-clotting.
Pine Bark Extract (Pinus Maritima, Pinus Haeda, Pinus Palustris, Pinus Pinaster)	V	A	3	3	Antioxidant; antiseptic. Rich in OPC (oligomeric proanthocyanidin) antioxidants. Source of bioflavaniods and organic acids. Anti-inflammatory and anti-viral properties.
Pistachio Nut Oil (Pistacia Vera)	V	M	2	3	Readily absorbed emollient oil. High in linoleic acid (30-35%).

Ingredient Name/INCI Name (Other Names in Parentheses)	Source	Purpose	S	LCR	Notes
Placental Extract	H, A	A, M	1	2	Available as the freeze-dried sterilized extract of human placenta, from full-term births. Also available from bovine (cattle) sources. It is a good source of RNA, DNA and vitamins. Believed to increase circulation and possibly increase cellular respiration.
Plantain Extract (Plantago Major)	V	A	2	3	Astringent; anti-inflammatory
Polyacrylamide	S	A	4-5	4-5	Solubilizer; lubricant; suspending agent. While polyacrylamide is relatively safe as normally used, if there is acrylamide monomer present in large amounts, these may be carcinogens. There should be less than 0.1%; the label will not indicate this data.
Polyethylene	S	Exf, A	3	2	The beads are used as an exfoliant. The emulsified material itself is generally used as film former.
Polyglyceryl-3 Laurate	V	M	3	3	Water-soluble emollient used in lipsticks, make-up and skin cream.
(Polyprepolymer 2) See "PPG-12/SMDI Copolymer"					
Polyquaternium-6, 22, 39, 47	S	A	3	3	Cationic conditioners and detanglers for hair and skin; film formers
Polyquaternium-7	S	A	3	3	Cationic conditioner; detangler for hair; film-former.
Polyquaternium-11	S	A	3	3	Film-forming hair fixative and hair conditioner. "Quat" type. Improves combability and manageability.
Polyquaternium-31	S	A, T	3	3-4	Skin conditioner; emulsion or suspension stabilizer
Polyquaternium-44	S	A	3	3	Primarily used as a conditioning polymer for shampoos. A cationic polymer that aids in combing and help reduce irritation on skin and scalp.

Ingredient Name/INCI Name (Other Names in Parentheses)	Source	Purpose	S	LCR	Notes
Polysorbate 20	V	E	2	2	Copolymerized sorbitol ester prepared from sorbitol (a sugar). Commonly used to solubilize oils, particularly perfume oils, in water-based products. Can help reduce irritation of the formula. (The most water soluble of the polysorbates)
Polysorbate 60	V	E	3	2	Copolymerized sorbitol ester prepared from sorbitol (a sugar). Commonly used to solubilize oils, particularly perfume oils, in water-based products. Can help reduce irritation of the formula.
Polysorbate 80 (Sorbitan Oleate)	V	E	3	2	Copolymerized sorbitol ester prepared from sorbitol (a sugar). Commonly used to solubilize oils, particularly perfume oils, in water-based products. Can help reduce irritation of the formula.
Polyvinyl Alcohol	S	T	3	3	Commonly used in peel off facial masks for its strong film-forming capability. The vinyl monomer content (if any) must be closely checked as it is potentially irritating and carcinogenic.
(Potassium Aluminum Sulfate) See "Alum"					
Potassium Chloride	M	T	1	3	Often used interchangeably with sodium chloride. (See "Sodium Chloride")
Potassium Cocoate	V	1	3	4	The name used for a soap formed from coconut oil fatty acids and potassium hydroxide (KOH), AKA "Caustic Potash." Can be very drying to the skin due to the alkaline pH. Can leave the typical "soap scum" residue when used with hard water.
Potassium Sorbate	S, V	P	2	3	Food grade preservative, more effective against yeasts and molds than it is against bacteria. Functions best below about pH 5.5.
Potato Starch (Solanum Tuberosum)	V	T	1	2	Thickener; absorbant

Ingredient Name/INCI Name (Other Names in Parentheses)	Source	Purpose	S	LCR	Notes
PPG					(Abbreviation for Polypropylene Glycol). As a prefix, it refers to a polymer of propylene oxide.
PPG-10, 20, etc., Cetyl Ether PPG-10, 20, etc., Stearyl Ether	S, V	M, SOL, A	3-4	3-4	Emollients and oil solubilizers used in a variety of products
PPG-12/SMDI Copolymer	S	A	2	2-3	Anti-irritant; also helps deposit and hold other ingredients in place. Used to slow and control the release of ingredients like vitamin A and AHAs and to reduce the likelihood of irritation. Has emollient properties and improves the "skin feel" of the product. Noncomedogenic.
Progesterone	A, S	A	4-5	3	A hormone listed as "reasonably anticipated to be (a) known carcinogen" in the "National Toxicology Program."
Propyl (Adjective only - not a molecule by itself)					The adjective "propyl" simply refers to that part of the molecule with a chain of 3 carbon atoms. It does not imply safety or lack thereof. (We listed this because of several consumer questions.)
Propylene Carbonate	S	SOL	3	3	Solvent for nail polish removers and to help form gels in lipsticks, deodorants, and mascaras.
Propylene Glycol (Propylene Glycol USP is the pharmaceutical grade, but is not required to be labeled as such on cosmetics.)	S	M, SOL	3	2 RO (generally) (At approx. 3%) 2-3 LV At approx. 4-8%) 3-4 LV (At approx. 8%) 4-5 LV	A food approved ingredient, that is used in personal care as an emollient, solubilizer or solvent. Widely used as an humectant, film plasticizer, and sometimes as a preservative (in concentrations above 15%). Tends to produce softer creams than glycerin or sorbitol. Propylene glycol can help increase the absorption of other, more irritating ingredients if improperly formulated and used in a high enough concentration. Often, it is used in low concentration (less than 1%) as a solvent to help other ingredients dissolve. It is also used to extract some plant materials. (Do not confuse with ethylene glycol - not the same)

Ingredient Name/INCI Name (Other Names in Parentheses)	Source	Purpose	S	LCR	Notes
Propylparaben (Propyl p-Hydroxybenzoate)	S	P	3-4	3-4	Preservative normally used at 0.2% or less. Particularly effective against yeasts. Parabens can be neutralized by nonionic emulsifiers.
(Provitamin B5) See "Panthenol"					
Pumice	M	Exf, AB	1	2	Volcanic stone/ash, ground and used as an abrasive or exfoliant.
PVM/MA Copolymer	S	A	3-4	3	Hair fixative used in hair sprays and gels. More flexible than PVP and less susceptible to humidity.
PVP (Polyvinylpyrrolidone)	S	A	3	2	Used to reduce the eye and skin irritation potential of other ingredients. Also used as a film former and hair fixative. Has barrier properties that can protect skin. Generally, too hygroscopic (absorbs water) for use as a hair spray fixative by itself. Also functions as a viscosity modifier in water-based systems. It is the polymer of 1-vinyl-2-pyrrolidone.
PVP/VA Coploymer	S	A	3-4	3	Hair fixative used in hair sprays and gels. More flexible than PVP and less susceptible to humidity.
Pycnogenol	V	O	3	3	Powerful antioxidant derived from pine bark
Pyridoxine - 3, 4 - dipalmitate	V, S	A	2	2	Source of vitamin B$_6$. Used as an anti-dandruff ingredient.
Pyridoxine Hydrochloride	V, S	A	1	2	One of the vitamins of the B$_6$ complex. Helps enhance mitotic activity of skin cells. Helps normalize and maintain healthy skin. Sometimes used to help control oil in skin and make-up products. A deficiency can lead to skin lesions.
Q					
(Q-10 Coenzyme) See "Coenzyme Q-10"			5	4 RO 5 LV	
Quaternium - 15	S	P	5		Preservative: believed to be a formaldehyde doner.

173

Ingredient Name/INCI Name (Other Names in Parentheses)	Source	Purpose	S	LCR	Notes
Quaternium - 18	S, A	A	3	3 RO 4 LV	"Quat" hair conditioner
Quaternium - 18 Hectorite & Quaternium - 18 Bentonite	S, M, A	T	3	3	Suspending agents; thickeners, particularly for oils. Also used as a barrier agent/skin protectant to protect skin against environmental abuse and contact dermatitis Helps sunscreens apply more evenly over the skin. (AKA "Quaternized" clays)
Quaternium - 26	S	A	3	3 RO	Hair conditioning "Quat," antistatic agent, emulsifier and film-former for hair setting products.
Quaternium - 27	S	A	3	3 RO 4 LV	"Quat" antistatic electricity agent and conditioner
Quaternium - 31 (Dicetyldimonium Chloride)	S	A	4	3-4 RO 4-5 LV	A hair and skin "Quat" type conditioner and antistatic agent
Quaternium - 52	S	A	3	3 RO 4 LV	Emulsifier; conditioner
Quaternium - 80	S	A	3	3 RO	A polymeric "Quat" used as a hair conditioner and antistatic agent. Compatible with anionic surfactants, unlike many "Quats."
Quaternium - 82	S	A, E	3	3 R 3-4 LV	A hair and skin "Quat" type conditioner and antistatic agent. Also used as a suspending agent in some foundation makeups.
Quaternium - 90 Bentonite	V, M	A, T	3	3	Suspending agent; thickener. Also used as a barrier agent/skin protectant to protect skin against environmental abuse and contact dermatitis. Helps sunscreens apply more evenly over the skin. (A "Quaternized" clay)

Ingredient Name/INCI Name (Other Names in Parentheses)	Source	Purpose	S	LCR	Notes
R					
(Rapeseed Oil) See "Canola Oil"					
Raspberry Leaf Extract (Rubas Idaeus)	V	A	2	2	Anti-irritant; anti-inflammatory. Contains ascorbic acid and isoflavones. Has astringent properties. Sometimes used to soothe reddened, irritated or burned skin.
Red Clover Leaf Extract	V	A	2	2	Source of phytoestrogens. Specifically biologically active estrogenic isoflavones. Commonly used internally in products to treat menopause.
Reishi Extract or Reishi Mushroom Extract (Ganoderma Lucidum)	V	A	1	2	Source of triterpene sterols and polysaccharides. Internally used for liver health and immune enhancing effects.
Resorcinol	S	A	4	5	Topical antiseptic and keratolytic (removes dead skin cells); anti-dandruff agent.
(Resveratrol)	V	A	2	2	A phytonutrient derived from grapeskin, with anti-inflammatory effects.
Retin A® (Vitamin A Acid; Tretinoin)	S	A	4	5	Brand name of Tretinoin, a member of the Vitamin A family. Makes skin very vulnerable to sunburn and sun damage. Highly effective peeling agent. (See "Retinoic Acid")
Retinoic Acid (Vitamin A Acid; Tretinoin)	V, A, S	A	4	5	For severe acne and also used as a skin peel. More likely to irritate than other forms of vitamin A.
Retinol (Vitamin A, Vitamin A Alcohol)	V, A, S	A, M, O	2	3	Occurs in animals, not in plants. (Plant carotenoids are converted into vitamin A by the liver.) Antioxidant and skin conditioner. (One of the fat-soluble vitamins, along with D, E & K.) Promotes healthy skin and skin cells; excellent in skin rejuvenating creams and lotions. Used in acne treatments and wound healing. There is evidence that vitamin A can enter the bloodstream via the skin if not formulated properly. Helps improve skin elasticity and normalize UV damaged skin. All forms of vitamin A can easily degrade if not properly formulated.

Ingredient Name/INCI Name (Other Names in Parentheses)	Source	Purpose	S	LCR	Notes
Retinyl Palmitate (Vitamin A Palmitate)	V, A, S	A, M, O	2	3	Source of vitamin A. Healing agent; antioxidant; acne treatment; used in the prophylaxis and treatment of photoageing and various skin disorders. Anti-keratinizing agent. When applied to the skin, much of it converts to Retinol. (See "Retinol")
Riboflavin (Vitamin B$_2$)	S,V	A	1	2	Minute amounts present in all plant and animal cells; required for various metabolic body processes. Can be used as a yellow colorant. Preserves integrity of the nervous system, skin and eyes. A deficiency can lead to dermatitis. Necessary for regeneration of the antioxidant glutathione. (Produced commercially as a fermentation product.)
Riboflavin -5' Phosphate Sodium	S, V	A	1	2	Enzyme form of vitamin B2 - more active and bioavailable. Can be used as a catalyst in tan accelerators.
Rice Amino Acids	V	M	2	2	Moisturizer; film former
Rice Bran Oil (Oryza Sativa)	V	M	2	3	Rich in vitamin E; has sunscreen properties
Rice Starch (Oryza Sativa)	V	T, A	1	2	Used as a skin soother and as a replacement for talc. Good absorbant. Ideal nutrient for bacteria - susceptible to contamination.
RNA (Ribonucleic Acid) and DNA (Deoxyribonucleic Acid)	A, S, H	A	2	3	Complex proteins found in every living cell, containing the cell's genetic code.
Rose Hips Oil (and extract) (Rosa Canina, Rosa Mosqueta)	V	M, A	2	3	The oil is rich in essential fatty acids (omega-3 and omega-6 fatty acids). The vitamin C content is in the aqueous extract, not in the oil. This oil is rich in linoleic acid (42-47%) and linolenic (30-35%).

Ingredient Name/INCI Name (Other Names in Parentheses)	Source	Purpose	S	LCR	Notes
Rosemary Extract (Rosmarinus Officinalis)	V	A, F, P	2	3	Antibacterial; astringent; fragrance. Applied externally as a treatment for excema, bruises and wounds. Also used as an antioxidant. Has some preservative properties. The actives are rosmarinic acid and carnosolic acid. The pure oil is a rubefacient.
Rosemary Oil (Rosmarinus Officinalis)	V	F	3	3-4 Depending on concentration	Essential oil for fragrances; aromatherapeutic oil. Rubefacient (causes reddening of the skin)
Rose Oil (Rosa Alba, Rosa Canina, Rosa Centifolia)	V	F	3	3- 4	Use in fragrances and in aromatherapy. Anti-inflammatory; calming; has mild astringent properties. Claimed to be an aphrodisiac. Rose oil N.F. is steam distilled from fresh flowers. The pure oil can be irritating to some people.
Rose Water (Rosa Alba, Rosa Canina, Rosa Centifolia)	V	F	2	3	Astringent; local tonic. Sometimes used on oily skin. Calming and anti-inflammatory properties.
Royal Jelly	A	M, A	1	2	Collected from beehives. Nutritive secretion of worker bees to feed the bee larvae and later, the queen bee. Contains proteins, carbohydrates, vitamins and minerals. Used in a variety of anti-aging, nourishing, moisturizing and rejuvenating formulas. High in B vitamins and nutrients. Claimed to rejuvenate skin and improve circulation when applied topically. Many of the claims are based on the vitamin B content.

S

Ingredient Name/INCI Name (Other Names in Parentheses)	Source	Purpose	S	LCR	Notes
Saccharomyces Lysate Yeast Extract or Saccharomyces Ferment	Yeast	A	2	3	Promotes wound healing; anti-inflammatory; soothing. Increases cleansing ability of shampoos. Used to reduce oiliness via enzymatic activity.

Ingredient Name/INCI Name (Other Names in Parentheses)	Source	Purpose	S	LCR	Notes
Safflower Oil (Carthamus Tinctorius)	V	M	1	2	High in polyunsaturated fatty acids, it has a unique feel and produces a different emulsion than other vegetable oils.
Sage Oil (Salvia Officinalis)	V	F	3	4	Stimulant; astringent; dandruff treatment; anti-inflammatory; antiseptic. Used as an antiperspirant - curbs excessive sweating. Insect repellant. Contains camphor. (Do not ingest the pure oil - high toxicity.)
St. John's Wort Extract (Hypericum Perforatum)	V	A	2	2	Used as an anti-inflammatory, phlebitis treatment, astringent and wound-healer. Sometimes used as a mild burn treatment. Can induce photosensitivity of the skin. Has antibacterial and antiviral properties. Internally used as an anti-depressant. Internally, can interfere with the activity of other drugs, such as HIV protease inhibitors and birth control formulas. Two of the actives are, hypericin and hyperforin.
Salicylic Acid	V, S	A	3	3 RO 3-4 LV 5 LV (At approx. 7%)	A beta hydroxy acid. Used to treat acne and other skin problems. Helps exfoliate skin. Occurs naturally in several plants, notably wintergreen leaves and the bark of sweet birch. Not for use in the sun - can cause sun sensitivity. Interestingly, it is restricted to 2% maximum in OTC drugs, but has no limit for cosmetic uses.
(Salt) See "Sodium Chloride"					
Sandalwood Oil (Santalum Album)	V	F	3	4	Essential oil used for fragrance blends or aromatherapy
Saponins	V	A, CL	3	3	Natural extracts used to increase foam in cleansing products
SD Alcohol 40 (A or B, 39, etc.)					This is ethanol that has been denatured (a bittering agent or the like is added to make it unfit for human ingestion). The number and/or letter is a code for which denaturant it contains. (See "Ethyl Alcohol" or appendix D)

Ingredient Name/INCI Name (Other Names in Parentheses)	Source	Purpose	S	LCR	Notes
Sea Kelp Extract See "Kelp" Also see "Seaweed Extract"					
Sea Salt	M	T	1	3	Salts from evaporated sea water, predominately sodium chloride, with many trace minerals.
Seaweed Extract [Sargassum Filipendula, Hypnea Musciformis, Gelidiela Acerosa, Fucus Vesiculosus (bladderwrack)]	V	A, M	2	2	Skin soother; moisturizer; anti-irritant; used to treat burns and insect bites. High in minerals, particularly iodine, depending on where it is harvested. Contains algin/sodium alginate - a mucopolysaccharide. Bladderwrack is used in anti-cellulite treatments.
Selenium	M	A	3-5 Depending on level used	4	Toxic at higher levels, it is an essential antioxidant and nutrient in trace quantities. Claimed to help with skin problems and other skin ailments. A component of one form of the important enzyme, glutathione peroxidase. Estimated safe internal daily intake is 50-200 mcg. A typical example of the concentration paradox - on one hand, selenium is important to human nutrition and may aid in preventing some cancers. On the other hand, it has a relatively low toxicity level. See bibliography reference No. 43 for more information.
Selenium Sulfide (Selenium Disulfide)	M	A	5	4	Used in anti-dandruff preparations. Listed as "reasonably anticipated to be a human carcinogen" by the National Toxicology Program.
Selenomethionine	M	A	2-4 Depending on dosage	3	Toxic at high levels, should be used only in trace amounts, where it functions as a powerful antioxidant. Source of bioavailable selenium, an essential nutrient. One of a group of trace metals needed for normal health. The toxicity is directly related to the level present. Dosage <1 milligram.
Sesame Oil (Sesamum Indicum)	V	M	2	2	Very light, versatile, vegetable oil used in skin care, hair care, nutritional supplements and pharmaceuticals. Extracted from the seed.
Shark Liver Oil	A	A	2	3	Source of vitamin A; skin protectant.

Ingredient Name/INCI Name (Other Names in Parentheses)	Source	Purpose	S	LCR	Notes
Shea Butter (Butyrospermum Parkii)	V	M	2	3	An occlusive type emollient. Anti-inflammatory; skin protectant. Has a mild sunscreen effect. Used traditionally as a healing agent, moisturizer and skin soother. (From the fruit kernel of an African tree.)
Shellac	A, V	A	3	3	A natural resin, used as a fixative in hair sprays and gels. Produces a hard, insoluble film. Sometimes used in lipsticks and eyeliners. Derived from insects.
Shiitake Extract or Shiitake Mushroom Extract (Lentinula Edodes)	V	A, O	1	2	The mushroom itself has a high beta glucan content, and contains anticancer and cholesterol reducing compounds.
Shikon Oil (Shikonin, Shicon, Lithospermum Officinale)	V	A, C	3	3	One of the active ingredients and principal component of "lithospermum." Moisturizer; skin treatment; has preservative properties. Used to treat a variety of skin problems, such as excema, acne, keratosis, etc. Some extracts are used as a color. (See "Lithospermum Extract")
Silica (Silicon Dioxide)	M	A, T	1	2	The more technical name for sand or quartz, the common form of the element silicon. Very finely ground silica is used as a drying agent. Helps powders maintain a free-flowing form by absorbing moisture. Do not breathe in the dust of the finely ground silica. Possible carcinogen in that type of exposure only.
Silicon	M	Not Used	2	2	A pure element (Si); second most abundant element on earth after oxygen. Does not occur free in nature; found as a component of silica (sand), silicates, clays or quartz.
Silicone(s)					A large group of silicon oxide polymers, with a multitude of uses. (See the individual silicones.)
Silk Amino Acids	A	A, M	2	2	Moisturizes and improves the skin feel of formulas. Derived from silk. Hair and skin conditioner; anti-irritant.

Ingredient Name/INCI Name (Other Names in Parentheses)	Source	Purpose	S	LCR	Notes
Silt (Russian Silt)	V, M	T, A	2	2	Skin conditioner; thickener for masks, etc. Source of trace minerals.
Silymarin See "Milk-Thistle Extract"					
Silver Nitrate	M	A	5	5	Astringent; antiseptic
Sodium Alginate	V	T, S	2	2	Anti-irritant; thickener (from seaweed)
Sodium Alpha Olefin Sulfonate (AOS)	V, S	CL	3-4	3-4 RO 4-5 LV	Anionic cleansing surfactant and emulsifier. Cleans well, even in hard water. "Sodium C$_{14-16}$ Olefin Sulfonate" is one type of this group.
Sodium Benzoate	V, S	P	3	3-4	Food approved preservative, usually used at less than 0.1%.
Sodium Bicarbonate (Baking Soda)	M	pH, AB	1	3	Used as an abrasive or as a means to raise the pH in certain products. The pH in water is about 8.3. Used as the effervescent agent in "fizzing" type bath salts.
Sodium Bisulfite	M	P	3-4	3-4 RO 4-5 LV	A stabilizer, used to help certain reactions from taking place in some formulas. Some people, especially those with asthma can have a serious reaction to foods containing sulfites. The FDA estimates that 1 in 100 persons are sulfite sensitive. We have not seen any evidence that this same reaction occurs when sulfites are used in skin care.
Sodium Borate (Borax)	M	A, pH, CI	4	3	Often used to neutralize beeswax to form an emulsion. (Forms sodium salts with the fatty acids in beeswax.) Less alkaline that the carbonates and has a mild detergent action when used in bath salts. More slow to dissolve and less effective as a water softener than the carbonates.
Sodium C$_{12-18}$ Alkyl Sulfate	V	CL	3	3-4	Anionic surfactant
Sodium C$_{14-16}$ Olefin Sulfonate (AOS)	V, S	CL	3-4	3-4 RO 4-5 LV	Anionic cleansing surfactant and emulsifier. Cleans well, even in hard water. A type of "Sodium Alpha Olefin Sulfonate"

Ingredient Name/INCI Name (Other Names in Parentheses)	Source	Purpose	S	LCR	Notes
Sodium Caproyl Lactate	V	E, A	3	3	Effective foam booster for amphoteric/betaine shampoos.
Sodium Carbomer	S	T	3	3-5	Carbomer, neutralized with sodium hydroxide. Thickener; stabilizer. (See "Carbomer")
Sodium Carbonate (Soda Ash) Sodium Carbonate Monohydrate Sodium Carbonate Decahydrate (Washing soda)	M	pH, AB	2	3	The pH in water is about 11.6. Effective water softener. Sometimes used in bath salts.
Sodium Carboxymethyl Cellulose (CMC)					See "Carboxymethyl Cellulose"
Sodium Carrageenan	V	T, S	2	2	A gum used to thicken and/or stabilize solutions and emulsions
Sodium Cetyl Sulfate	V	CL, E	3	3	Cleanser; emulsifier
Sodium Chloride (Common Salt; Sea Salt)	M	T	1	3	Used to thicken the viscosity of shampoos and bath gels. Also used as an inexpensive filler for bath salts and dry bubble baths. Does not soften water. Interferes with soap lathering.
Sodium Citrate	M, V	pH	2	3	Used to adjust the pH in various products and/or as a buffering agent
Sodium Cocamphoacetate	V	CL	3	3	Mild cleansing amphoteric surfactant; foam booster; has conditioning properties
Sodium Cocosulfate	V	CL	3	3-4	Surfactant; cleanser
Sodium Cocoyl Glutamate	V	CL	3	2	Made from natural fatty acids and L-glutamic amino acid Very mild and biodegradable. Compatible with many cationics, unlike most anionic cleansers.
Sodium Cocoyl Isethionate	V	CL	3	3	Lower foaming than the lauryl sulfate cleansers. Usually used in "bar" form because it can be hydrolyzed in solution. Formed by "connecting" fatty acids directly to a surfactant without going through the fatty alcohol stage.

Ingredient Name/INCI Name (Other Names in Parentheses)	Source	Purpose	S	LCR	Notes
Sodium Cocoyl Methyltaurate	V	CL	3	3	A mild cleansing surfactant, made from coconut fatty acids.
Sodium Cocoyl Sarcosinate	V	CL	3	3	A mild cleansing surfactant, made from coconut fatty acids. Mild, biodegradable, with low toxicity.
Sodium Dehydroacetate	S	P	3-4	3-4 RO 4-5 LV	Fungicide; bactericide. Has some food-approved uses.
Sodium Hyaluronate	V, A	M, A	1	2	Sodium salt of hyaluronic acid. (See "Hyaluronic Acid")
Sodium Hydrosulfite	M	A	3-5	3 RO 3-5 LV	Reducing agent to help prevent certain chemical reactions from occurring within finished products.
Sodium Hydroxymethylglycinate	S, V	P	3	4	Preservative, milder than most.
Sodium Glutamate	V, S	M, A	3	3	The sodium salt of L-glutamic acid (an amino acid).
Sodium Lactate	V, S	M	2	3	An humectant with superior moisture uptake effects. Occurs naturally in the skin.
Sodium Laureth Sulfate	V, S	CL	3	3 RO	One of the most commonly used surfactants. An ethoxylated (milder) version of sodium lauryl sulfate. As the amount of ethoxylation increases, viscosity decreases and mildness increases. An ethoxylated lauryl alcohol is used instead of the lauryl alcohol used to make sodium lauryl sulfate.
Sodium Lauroamphoacetate	V	CL	3	3	Amphoteric, mild cleanser
Sodium Lauroyl Sarcosinate	V	CL	3	3	Surfactant derived from the amino acid "sarcosin" and lauryl alcohol. More substantive to hair than the lauryl or laureth sulfates. Mild, biodegradable, with low toxicity.
Sodium Lauryl Sulfate	V, S	CL	3	3-4 RO 4-5 LV Depending on concentration used	The classic fatty alcohol sulfate surfactant. Strongest cleanser (at equal concentration) of the lauryl sulfate group. Excellent foamer. Produces a high viscosity. It can be over-drying or irritating if used at too high a level and/or improperly formulated. As we have noted before – the percentage level is one key to determining safety and irritation. (See pages 4-8, and 19-21)

Ingredient Name/INCI Name (Other Names in Parentheses)	Source	Purpose	S	LCR	Notes
Sodium Lauryl Sulfoacetate	V	CL	3	3	Relatively mild cleanser; low toxicity; excellent foaming characteristics; yields good viscosity. Sometimes used as a soap replacement for individuals sensitive to soaps. Biodegradable; approved for use in dental products.
Sodium Metabisulfite	M	P	4	3-4 RO 4-5 LV	Preservative; anti-oxidant
Sodium Myreth Sulfate	V	CL	3	3	See "Sodium Laureth Sulfate" (Myristyl alcohol is used instead of lauryl alcohol).
Sodium PCA (Sodium 2-pyrrolidone-5-carboxylate)	V, S	M	2	2	PCA is a natural component of human skin. Excellent humectant and moisturizer at concentrations above about 2%. Usually made from plant-derived glucose.
Sodium Polystyrene Sulfonate	S	A	3	3 RO 4 LV	A hair conditioner and styling aid that also claims (in shampoos) to help remove cationic conditioner build-up on the hair. It is said to accomplish this via an anionic charge on the molecule itself, and in a more mild fashion than anionic shampoos.
Sodium Pyrithione	M, S	A	3-4	4 RO 5 LV	Anti-microbial; preservative; anti-dandruff agent
Sodium Sesquicarbonate	M	A	3	3	Used as the main ingredient in many bath salts. Effective water softener. PH about 9.8 (1% solution). Reasonably mild to the skin.
Sodium Silicate	M	A	2	3-4	Skin firmer; source of silicon
Sodium Stearate	V, A	E	2	3	Sodium salt of stearic acid. Commonly used to solidify glycerin or harden "stick" type products. Thickener.
Sodium Stearoyl Lactylate	V	E, M	3	3	Humectant; emulsifier; has some food-approved uses.
Sodium Sulfate	M	T	3	3	Sometimes used as an inexpensive filler for bath salts and dry bubble bath products.

Ingredient Name/INCI Name (Other Names in Parentheses)	Source	Purpose	S	LCR	Notes
Sodium Sulfite	M	A, P	4	3-4 RO 4-5 LV	Reducing agent. Sometimes used in hair relaxers or permanent waxes. Also used to retard some reactions in certain formulas. Used as a stabilizer. (See "Sodium Bisulfite")
Soluble Collagen	A	M	2	3	Film-former, from partially hydrolyzed animal tissue. Lubricates and moisturizes skin and hair. (A protein)
Sorbic Acid	V, S	P	3	3	Organic acid; food approved preservative, usually used at about 0.1% or less. Not effective above approximately pH 5.6.
Sorbitan Isostearate	V	E	2	3	A liquid sorbitan ester used as a wetting agent and emulsifier. A "water in oil" emulsifier.
Sorbitan Oleate	V	E	2	2	Nonionic solubilizer and emulsifier. A "water in oil" emulsifier.
Sorbitan Stearate (Sorbitan Monostearate)	V	E	2	2	Nonionic solubilizer and emulsifier. A "water in oil" emulsifier.
Sorbitan Trioleate	V	E	2	3	Emollient; emulsifier
Sorbitol	V	M, A	1	2	Humectant; sweetener that occurs naturally in many berries. A current common commercial source is beets. Used as a sweetener and taste/mouth feel enhancer in toothpastes.
Soya Liposomes	V	A	2-4	2-4	The liposome shell itself is very safe. The overall safety depends on what is in the liposome. See "Liposome" in the "Terms" section of this book.
Soya Sterol	V	E, M	2	2	Excellent natural emulsifier and emollient (from soybeans). A recent study shows them to have anti-inflammatory and conditioning properties. Internally, studies indicate Soya Sterols may help lower cholesterol.
Soybean Oil (Glycine Soya)	V	M	1	3	Light vegetable oil used in skin care, nutritional supplements and pharmaceutical delivery systems.

Ingredient Name/INCI Name (Other Names in Parentheses)	Source	Purpose	S	LCR	Notes
Soy Isoflavones	V	A	3	3	Phytoestrogen source from soybean molasses. Non-steroidal, weaker than natural estrogens. Not stored in the body. Antioxidant properties. Believed to help the immune system. Internally, also used in treatment of diabetes.
Spearmint Oil (Mentha Viridis)	V	F	2	4	Used primarily as a fragrance or flavor. Unlike peppermint oil, it does not contain menthol. Taken internally, soothing to the stomach.
Spermaceti (Synthetic Spermaceti)	A,S	T, E	3	3	Originally from the oil of the sperm whale, it is no longer for sale in the United States. Synthetic Spermaceti is now used in the United States. See "Cetyl Esters"
Squalane	V, A, S	M	2	3	Shark liver and olive oil are the primary sources. Excellent moisturizer similar to ingredients in natural skin oils. Light, oily substance also used as a skin lubricant. (Saturated hydrocarbon)
Squalene	V, A, S	M	3	4	Unsaturated hydrocarbon, from olive oil, wheat germ oil or shark liver oil. A component of human sebum (skin oil). Emollient and lubricant.
Stearalkonium Bentonite	S, V, A, M	T, S	3	3	Suspending agents; thickeners. Also used as a barrier agent/skin protectant to protect skin against environmental abuse and contact dermatitis. Helps sunscreens apply more evenly over the skin. (A "Quaternized" clay)
Stearalkonium Chloride	S, V, A	A	3	3-4	Hair conditioner; antistatic electricity ingredient
Stearamide DEA	V	E	3	4	Thickener; emulsifier
Stearamide MEA	V	E	3	3	Thickener; opacifier; emulsifier
Stearamidopropyl Dimethylamine	S, V	E, A	3-4	3-4	Hair conditioner; cationic emulsifier with enhanced substantivity to skin. Lower irritation than normal quaternary conditioners. Unlike most "Quats" it is compatible with anionic surfactants in shampoos. Improves "wet-combing" and claimed to improve hair "volume."

Ingredient Name/INCI Name (Other Names in Parentheses)	Source	Purpose	S	LCR	Notes
Steareth-2	V	E	2	4	Nonionic emulsifier from stearic acid. Most oil soluble of the group.
Steareth-4 through 100	V	E	2	3	Nonionic emulsifiers from stearic acid. Becomes more water soluble as the number increases.
Stearic Acid	V, A	E	2	3	A natural fatty acid, probably the most common in creams and lotions. It usually is a mixture of fatty acids, predominately stearic acid. Often neutralized with triethanolamine or sodium hydroxide to form a soap type cream emulsion - the traditional "vanishing cream." Because they are soaps, these creams generally have a higher pH of about 6.5 - 8.0.
Stearyl Alcohol (Octadecanol)	V, S	E	2	2	Fatty alcohol. An emulsifier and thickener derived from stearic acid. Has emollient properties.
Stearyl Dimethicone (Alkyl Modified Silicone)	M	M	3	3	Dimethicone, modified by the addition of an alkyl group, to improve viscosity of the final product, skin feel, "spreadability" and/or improve color pigment dispersion.
Stearyl Octanoate	V	M, E	3	3	
Stearoyl Stearate	V	E	2	2	Emollient; emulsifier; opacifier; from stearic acid. (A solid material at room temperature.)
Sugar Cane Extract (Saccharum Officinarium)	V	A	3	3-4	Usually used as a natural source of glycolic acid. The name itself does not tell you exactly what is extracted. Could be only sugar, for example.
Sulfur (Brimstone)	M	A	4 (At >1%) 3 (At< 1%)	3-4 RO 4-5 LV	Antibacterial, antifungal, and anti-acne ingredient. It is a keratolytic agent. Used in some oily skin products at low levels. The percentage is important. We recommend less than 1% for external use. Do not ingest.
(Sulisobenzone) See "Benzophenone-4"					

Ingredient Name/INCI Name (Other Names in Parentheses)	Source	Purpose	S	LCR	Notes
Sunflower Oil (Helianthus Annuus)	V	M	1	3	A mixture of fatty acids used as an emollient (rich in omega-6 fatty acids).
Sunflower Seed Extract	V	M, A	2	3	Vegetable ceramides, similar to natural human ceramides, used to help maintain the intercellular moisture barrier of the stratum corneum. Helps keep skin flexible and prevents environmental attacks on the skin. Source is sunflowers. (See "Ceramides")
(Sweet Almond Oil) See "Almond Oil - Sweet"					
Synthetic Beeswax	S	E, M	3	3	A synthetic beeswax, that is used to avoid the batch to batch variation of natural beeswax.
(Synthetic Spermaceti) See "Cetyl Esters"					
T					
Talc (Talcum)	M	A	2	3	Used in many powder products such as face powder. As a dusting or "baby" powder, some inhalation concerns should be noted. Avoid breathing the powder. In water-based products, it is safe and used as a thickener and to improve "skin feel." Provides "slip" and a smooth feel to the product. Do not use on open wounds or inflammation. It is important to make certain that the material used is of the asbestos -free grade. There are a large number of varieties available. Do not use feminine hygiene products containing talc.
Tallow	A	M	2	3	Beef or sheep fat. Used as an emollient and/or ointment base.
Tangerine Oil (Citrus Tangerina)	V	F	2	2-3 RO / 3-4 LV Depending on level used	Used as a flavor or fragrance. Has astringent properties.

Ingredient Name/INCI Name (Other Names in Parentheses)	Source	Purpose	S	LCR	Notes
Tartaric Acid (L-Tartaric Acid	V	A	2	4	Alpha hydroxy fruit acid, found in many fruits, particularly during grape fermentation. Much of what is sold today is a by-product of the wine industry.
(TEA) See "Triethanolamine"					
TEA-Carbomer	S	T	3	4	Thickener. Reaction product of triethanolamine and carbomer. (See "Carbomer")
TEA-Cocoyl Glutamate	V	CL	3	2-3	Very mild anionic cleansing surfactant, derived from coconut fatty acids and glucose. Very mild and biodegradable compared to many other cleansers.
TEA-Cocoyl-Hydrolyzed Animal Protein, and TEA Cocoyl-Hydrolyzed Collagen	A	A, CL	2	2	Protein based anionic surfactants with conditioning properties. Mild; low irritation.
TEA-Dodecylbenzenesulfonate (and other Benzene Sulfonates)	S	CL	3	4	Strong cleanser; can over-clean and dry hair. Higher likelihood of irritation than many other cleansers. Not acceptable for bubble baths. Not as biodegradable as many other surfactant cleansers.
TEA-Laureth Sulfate (TLES)	V, S	CL	3	3	Mild cleansing surfactant
TEA-Lauryl Sulfate (TLS)	V, S	CL	3	3-4	Alkyl sulfate, milder than sodium lauryl sulfate (SLS). Produces a rich lather in cleansers. Like all alkyl sulfates, has a tendency to over-clean in high concentrations and must be properly formulated. Produces less viscosity and has a lower "cloud point" than SLS.
TEA-Stearate	V	E	2	3	Soap type emulsifier formed from stearic acid, neutralized with triethanolamine.
Tea Tree Oil (Melaleuca Alternifolia)	V	A, P	3	3-4	Germicide, fungicide and antiseptic, from the leaves of an Australian tree. Used to treat burns, abrasions, insect bites, athlete's foot and other conditions. Germicidal properties due to terpinen-4-ol (terpene hydrocarbon), which is about 35-45% of the oil. One supplier encapsulates it in cyclodextrin to protect it against oxidation. Do not ingest.

189

Ingredient Name/INCI Name (Other Names in Parentheses)	Source	Purpose	S	LCR	Notes
Tetrahydrodiferuloyl Methane	V	0	3	2	Antioxidant, from turmeric (spice) (AKA: Tetrahydrocuminoids)
Tetrasodium EDTA	M	P, A	3	3	See "Disodium EDTA" – same uses
Thiamine Hydrochloride	S, V, A	A	2	2	Water soluble form of vitamin B1. Occurs in plants and animal tissue. Keeps mucous membranes healthy, promotes normal growth and development, and is important in many reactions that take place within the body.
Thioctic Acid					See "Alpha Lipoic Acid"
Thioglycolic Acid (Mercaptoacetic and Ammonium Thioglycolate (Used in "Alkaline" perms, about pH 9+), and MEA-Thioglycolate (used in perms about pH 8 - 9), and Glyceryl Thioglycolate (used in "acid" perms about pH 6 - 8)	S	A	5	5	Used in many hair straighteners and cold wave solutions. (A "reducing agent.") The thioglycolate breaks the sulfide bonds in hair, the hair is reshaped, then the bonds are reestablished by use of a neutralizer - usually peroxide. Also used in depilatories to remove hair. Can damage hair if misused, and can irritate skin.
Thyme Oil (Thymus Vulgaris)	V	A, F	3	4	An essential oil used as a fragrance or astringent. Topical antiseptic; used for treating rashes. In the bath, the oil is used to relieve tired muscles and exhaustion. Contains thymol. (Do not ingest the pure oil - high toxicity.)
Thymol	V, S	A, P	4	5	Can be obtained from thyme oil. Anti-fungal; preservative; antiseptic against fungi, bacteria and some parasites. Used as a flavor ingredient and a denaturant in one type of "specially denatured" ethanol. (See "SD Alcohol")

Ingredient Name/INCI Name (Other Names in Parentheses)	Source	Purpose	S	LCR	Notes
Titanium Dioxide	M, S	A, C	2	2	Whitener; topical protectant; sunscreen. Used in make-up as a whitener and opacifier. Greater "whitening" or covering power than zinc oxide. Non-toxic; generally inert.
Tocopherol (Vitamin E)	V, S	A, M, O	1	2	The natural form is d-a tocopherol. The synthetic is dl-a tocopherol. Used in the treatment and prevention of various skin disorders and photoageing. Antioxidant; helps protect cell membranes; skin healing agent. Also functions as an antioxidant in the product to prevent rancidity. Internally, helps prevent arterial plaque and platelet aggregation. Helps prevent nitrosamine formation in personal care products. d-a tocopherol is natural vitamin E, usually derived from soybeans. It is an excellent skin moisturizer and healing agent, but tends to be somewhat "greasy" feeling at concentrations above about 5,000 IU/oz. Excellent skin healing agent, occlusive type moisturizer and anti-ageing antioxidant. Protects against UV damage, ozone and keeps skin smooth and flexible. The amount in the body can be reduced by stress.
Tocopheryl Acetate	V, S	A, M	2	2	An ester form of vitamin E. dl-a-tocopheryl acetate is synthetic, d-a tocopheryl acetate is naturally derived. More stable than tocopherol. (See "Tocopherol")
Tocopheryl Linoleate	V	A, M	1	2	Intensive skin moisturizer, protectant and healer. One of our most highly recommended ingredients to keep skin soft and flexible. Repairs/restores the intracellular moisture barrier of the skin. Keeps the stratum corneum flexible. Antioxidant. (See "Tocopherol")
Tocopheryl Nicotinate	V	A	3	3-4	Circulation stimulator. Anti-inflammatory and source of vitamin E. (See "Tocopherol")
Toluene	S, P	SOL	5	5	Known irritant
Tragacanth Gum (Astragalus Gummifer)	V	T	2	2	A plant derived complex mixture of polysaccharides, used as a film former and viscosity builder in lotions and gels. Stable from pH 3.5 to 8.5, most stable at pH 5.

Ingredient Name/INCI Name (Other Names in Parentheses)	Source	Purpose	S	LCR	Notes
Tri Alkyl Citrate Tri C₁₂₋₁₃ Alkyl Citrate Tri C₁₄₋₁₅ Alkyl Citrate	V, P	M, SOL	3	3	Emollient; color pigment carrier and disperser
Tribehenin (Glyceryl Tribehenate)	V	T	3	3	Gellant; thickening agent; suspending agent. A wax that also provides emolliency and gloss. Manufactured from glycerides and fatty acids. (Triester of glycerin and behenic acid)
Triclosan	S	P	4	4-5	Often used in soaps, cleansers, lotions and deodorants for its antibacterial properties. Also used as a preservative. Normally used at 0.1 - 1.0% in personal care products.
Trideceth – 3, 5, etc.	V, S	E	3	3	Emulsifiers
Triethanolamine (TEA)	S	pH	3	4	Used to raise the pH of a product and/or neutralize acidic ingredients. It is a mildly alkaline substance and is often used in place of sodium hydroxide to neutralize soaps or other products. The resulting product is generally more mild than if sodium hydroxide was used.
Triethyl Citrate	V, S	A	3	3	Perfume solvent; plasticizer; deodorant, made from citric acid and ethanol.
Trilaurin (Glyceryl Trilaurate)	V	A	3	3	Lipid similar to those found in the skin
Trimethylsiloxysilicate	M, S	M	3	3	Silicone type moisture barrier agent
Trimethylsilyl Trimethylsiloxysalicate	M, S	A	3	3-4	Produces salicylic acid in a more controlled fashion, to help reduce irritation. Typically used in acne products.
Trisodium Ethylenediamine Disuccinate	S	A	3	3	Chelating agent used to replace EDTA type chelates. Claimed to be more biodegradable than EDTA compounds.
Tyrosine (L-Tyrosine)	A, V	A	2	3	An amino acid believed to play an important part in tanning (melanin formation in the skin). The amount of tyrosine in the skin controls the melanin (pigmentation) formation. Often used in tanning accelerators. Internally, the body uses Tyrosine to make the neurochemicals seratonin and dopamine.

Ingredient Name/INCI Name (Other Names in Parentheses)	Source	Purpose	S	LCR	Notes
U					
Ubiquinone					See "Coenzyme Q-10"
Ultramarine Blue	M	C	4	4	From lapis lazuli originally, now prepared from minerals reacted at high temperatures.
Ultramarine Green	M	C	4	4	Inorganic color pigment, created by means of high temperature reaction.
Ultramarine Pink	M	C	4	4	Inorganic color pigment, created by means of high temperature reaction.
Ultramarine Red	M	C	4	4	Inorganic color pigment, created by means of high temperature reaction.
Ultramarine Violet	M	C	4	4	Made from ultramarine blue
Undecylenic Acid	S	P	4	4-5	Preservative: antimicrobial
Urea (Carbamide)	S	M, A	3	4	Excellent humectant and moisturizer; antiseptic; treatment for dermatitis. Helps promote wound healing. Occasionally, we are asked if it comes from urine. It does not. Can be a keratolytic at high concentrations (about 20%).
Urea Peroxide	S	A	4	5	Oxidizer. Used as a neutralizer in cold waving.
Usinic Acid	V, S	P	4	4-5	Preservative: antimicrobial (can be obtained from lichen plant).
(Uva Ursi) See "Bearberry Extract"					
V					
VA/Crotonates Copolymer	S	A	3-4	3-4	Film forming hair set resin
VA/VP Copolymer					See "PVP/VA Copolymer"

Ingredient Name/INCI Name (Other Names in Parentheses)	Source	Purpose	S	LCR	Notes
Valerian (Root) Extract (Valariana Officinalis, Valeriana Wallichii)	V	A	2	2	Antioxidant properties. Active ingredient is valerenic acid. Natural sedative when taken internally. Calmative; muscle relaxant. Has been used as a flavoring in root beer.
Vanilla Extract (Vanilla Planifolia, Vanilla Tahitensis)	V	F	1	3	Used as a flavor and/or fragrance. Used in aromatherapy.
Vinegar	V	A, pH	1	3-4	Astringent; acidic solution to lower the pH. Vinegar is a weak solution of acetic acid in water.
(Vitamin A) See "Retinol" and "Retinyl Palmitate"					
(Vitamin B1) See "Thiamine Hydrochloride"					
(Vitamin B2) See "Riboflavin"					
(Vitamin B3) See "Niacin" and "Niacinamide"					
(Vitamin B5) See "Panthenol" and "Pantothenic Acid"					
(Vitamin B6) See "Pyridoxine Hydrochloride"					
(Vitamin B12) See "Cyanocobalamin"					

Ingredient Name/INCI Name (Other Names in Parentheses)	Source	Purpose	S	LCR	Notes
(Vitamin C) See "Ascorbic Acid"					
(Vitamin D) See "Cholecalciferol" and "Ergocalciferol"					
(Vitamin E) See "Tocopherol"					
(Vitamin F - unofficial) (Essential Fatty Acids)					A term used for a group of fatty acids - particularly linolenic acid - believed essential to cell wall integrity, general human nutrition and healthy skin. Good sources include wheat germ oil, borage oil and evening primrose oil.
(Vitamin H) See "Biotin"					
(Vitamin K) See "Phytonadione"					
W					
Walnut Shell Powder (Juglans Regia, Juglans Mandshurica)	V	Exf, AB	1	1	Ground walnut shells; exfoliant
Water	M	SOL	1	1	Usually refers to "deionized water" in the world of cosmetics. This is the proper labeling name for all types of water - purified, deionized, demineralized, spring water, aqueous extract solvent, etc. Even water can be irritating, albeit mildly, under the right circumstances.
Wheat Amino Acids	V	A	1	3	Moisturizer; hair and skin conditioner

Ingredient Name/INCI Name (Other Names in Parentheses)	Source	Purpose	S	LCR	Notes
Wheat Germamidopropyl Betaine	V	CL	2	3	Very mild betaine type surfactant, made from wheat germ oil fatty acids. Has some light conditioning properties.
Wheat Germ Extract (Triticum Vulgare)	V	A	1	2-3	Depending on what it is extracted with, it may contain vitamin E, minerals and/or B vitamins. The aqueous extract for example, will not contain the oil soluble vitamin E, but may contain minerals and the B vitamins.
Wheat Germ Glycerides	V	M	2	2	Mixture of glycerides produced by transesterification of wheat germ oil. Emollient; skin lubricant; anti-irritant.
Wheat Germ Oil (Triticum Vulgare)	V	M, A	1	2-3	Sometimes used as a natural source of vitamin E because of the naturally high content of tocopherols. A source of gamma linoleic acid, one of the "essential fatty acids" needed for healthy skin. Natural source of vitamins E, A, D and octacosanol (from wheal kernel).
Wheat Starch (Triticum Vulgare)	V	M, T	1	2-3	Absorbant; skin soother
White Willow Bark Extract (Salix Alba)	V	A	2	3	Natural source of pain-relieving salicylates, which act as analgesics, astringents and antiseptics. Used to treat wounds and eczema, and to stop bleeding. Good for acne. One active ingredient is called "salicin."
Wild Yam Extract (Dioscorea Composita, Dioscorea Villosa)	V	A	2	3	Used as a source pf phytoestrogens in female directed formulas. The amount of yam is not important. Try to determine the active saponegin content (diosgenin). Do not confuse D. composita with other species of yam that may not contain a high level of phytoestrogens. These natural compounds can be laboratory altered to produce steroid hormones. There is no study, to our knowledge, that proves that these natural diosgenin compounds in wild yam are transformed to steroidal compounds in the human body when applied in creams or taken internally. Also has anti-inflammatory properties.
Wintergreen Oil (Gaultheria Procumbens)	V, S	A, F	4-5	4-5	Natural essential oil. Used for fragrance, flavor and/or cooling effect on the skin. Also used as a counterirritant. The herb is a source of methyl salicylate. The synthetic oil is generally almost pure methyl salicylate. (See "Methyl Salicylate".)

Ingredient Name/INCI Name (Other Names in Parentheses)	Source	Purpose	S	LCR	Notes
Witch Hazel Extract (Hamamelis Virginiana)	V	A	3	3	Astringent qualities probably due to natural tannin and/or the alcohol content. Antibacterial because it is in about 20% alcohol (ethanol or isopropanol). The herb itself is an anti-inflammatory. Vasoconstrictor; oily skin treatment.
X					
Xanthan Gum	V	T, S	1	2	Thickening and emulsion stabilizing polysaccharide gum approved for food use. Produced by fermentation of a carbohydrate.
Xanthene	V, S	O	1-2	2	Antioxidant, usually derived from vegetable sources
Xylene (Dimethylbenzene)	P	SOL	5	5	Aromatic hydrocarbon solvent
Xylitol	V	A	3	3	Sweetener made from xylose, a natural sugar
Y					
Yarrow Extract (Achillea Millefolium)	V	A	2	3-4	Related to chamomile; antiseptic; astringent; tonic and stimulant herb. High in flavonoids. Traditionally used in ointments for healing or stopping the bleeding of wounds. Anti-inflammatory. Some species contain azulene.
(Yeast Beta Glucan) See "Beta Glucan"					
Yeast Extract	V	M, A	3	3	Usually dried yeast cells of saccharomyces. Antioxidant; moisturizer; vitamin source; healing agent.
Ylang-Ylang Oil (Cananga Odorata)	V	F	3	4	Essential oil used in the manufacture of fragrances, or as a pure oil in aromatherapy.
Yohimbe	V	A	3	3	Contains alkaloids believed to be sexual function enhancers. Acts as a vasoconstrictor. Usually taken internally for these effects. (From the bark of the tree)

Ingredient Name/INCI Name (Other Names in Parentheses)	Source	Purpose	S	LCR	Notes
Yucca Extract (Yucca Vera, Yucca Aloifolia, Yucca Brevifolia-Joshua Tree)	V	CL, A	2	3	Usually used as a foaming agent and/or very mild cleanser due to high natural saponin content. From the yucca cactus of the American Southwest. Skin soother.
Z					
Zinc Gluconate and Zinc Citrate	M	A	3	3	Water soluble sources of zinc, necessary for proper skin health. Zinc is a necessary nutrient. It plays an important role in body enzymes and the synthesis of DNA and RNA. Crucial to normal bone growth. Possibly crucial to activation of Vitamin A in the eye. Used in common cold treatments.
Zinc Oxide	M	C, A	2	2	Sunscreen; whitening agent and skin protectant. Provides a mechanical barrier for the skin. Very occlusive. A basic ingredient of many "ointments" and other water-free creams. Non-toxic. Used in therapy of minor skin irritations. Has been used in place of hydrocortisone to soothe and "calm" irritated skin.
Zinc Pyrithione	M	A	4	3-4 RO 4-5 LV	Antidandruff ingredient; antimicrobial
Zinc Stearate	V, S, M	E	3	3	Emulsifier and source of zinc. Also an astringent and topical protective (barrier coating). Provides "smoothness" and adhesion to eye shadows. Also can provide water repellency. Anti-caking agent.
Zinc Sulfate	M	A	3	3-4	Source of zinc. Astringent. Believed to be most absorbable form of zinc. Internally, zinc is an essential mineral needed for DNA and RNA synthesis, bone formation, healthy skin and eyes, the immune system, male sexual function, and many other body functions. While zinc is present in plants, other ingredients such as tannins and some organic acids inhibit absorption. This can necessitate supplementation for vegetarians.
Zirconium Chloride (Zirconium Oxychloride) (Zirconyl Chloride)	M, S	A	4	5	Antiperspirant active ingredient

Appendix A
Sources of Information

I.   For the safety and chemical structure of many common
     ingredients:
     A.   *The Merck Index*; Eleventh Edition, Merck & Co., Inc.,
          Rahway, NJ, U.S.A., 1989.
     B.   *The International Cosmetic Ingredient Dictionary and Hand-
          book*, Published by The Cosmetics, Toiletries and Fra-
          grance Association, Inc., Washington, DC, Eighth Edition,
          2000.
     C.   *CIR* (Cosmetic Ingredient Review), 1101 17th St., N.W.,
          Suite 310, Washington, DC, 20036-4702
          Phone: (202) 331-0651; cirinfo@cir-safety.org

II. For formulation of cosmetic products:
     A.   Alexander, P., et al., *Harry's Cosmeticology*, New York,
          NY, Chemical Publishing, 2000.
     B.   de NaVarre, M.G., *The Chemistry and Manufacture of Cos-
          metics—Volume IV*, Orlando, FL, Continental Press, 1975.
     C.   Jellinek, S.J., Dr., *Formulation and Function of Cosmetics*,
          New York, NY, John Wiley & Sons Inc., 1970.

III. For the latest cosmetic research:
     A.   *Global Cosmetic Industry Magazine*, Duluth, MN,
          Advanstar Communications, Inc.
     B.   *Happi Magazine (Household and Personal Products Indus-
          try)*, Ramsey, NJ, Rodman Publishing Corporation.
     C.   *Soap and Cosmetics Magazine*, New York, NY, Chemical
          Week Associates.

IV. Cosmetic companies with 800 numbers and laboratories:
     A.   Earth Science, Inc.
          475 N. Sheridan Street
          Corona, CA 92880
          Phone: (800) 222-6720; www.earthscienceinc.com.
     B.   Terrapin Outdoor Systems
          P.O. Box 40339
          Santa Barbara, CA 93140
          Phone: (805) 682-6250; info@goturtle.com.

C. Kerstin Florian, Inc.
    15375 Barranca Parkway
    Suite A-104
    Irvine, CA 92618
    Phone (949) 753-0225
    E-mail kerstin@kerstinflorianinc.com

V. Websites:
    A. American Chemical Society: www.acs.org
    B. Allured Bookstore: www.store.yahoo.com/allured
    C. California Air Resources Board: www.arb.ca.gov/themis
    D. Cosmetic and Toiletries Magazine: www.cosmtoil.com
    E. Cosmetics, Toiletry and Fragrance Association:
        www.ctfa.org
    F. Food and Drug Law Institute: www.fdli.org
    G. Global Cosmetics: www.globalcosmetic.com
    H. National Toxicology Program:
        ntp-server.niehs.nih.gov/Main_pages/NTP.
    I. Society of Cosmetic Chemists (global): www.scs.co.uk
    J. Society of Cosmetic Chemists (USA): www.scconline.org
    K. U.S. Library of Congress: www.lcweb.loc.gov
    L. U.S. Pharmacopeia: www.usp.org
    M. U.S. Food and Drug Administration (FDA):
        www.FDA.gov.

Appendix B: Oils and Fats[1]

	ALMOND	AVOCADO	CASTOR	COCONUT	CORN	COTTON-SEED	OLIVE	PEANUT	PERSIC	RICE BRAN	SAF-FLOWER	SEASAME	SOYBEAN	SUN-FLOWER	WALNUT
C 8:0 CAPRYLIC				5 - 9											
C 10:0 CAPRIC				4 - 10											
C 12:0 LAURIC	0.2 MAX			44 - 52											
C 14:0 MYRISTIC	1.5 MAX	0.1 - 2.1		13 - 21	1 MAX	0.5 - 2.0	0.1 - 1.2	< 0.2		< 1	< 1	< 0.5	< 0.5	< 0.1	
C 16:0 (CETYL) PALMITIC	3 - 9	7.5 - 25	0.8 - 1.8	8 - 11	8 - 19	17 - 29	7 - 16	6 - 15.5	2.4	12 - 18	2 - 10	7 - 12	7 - 12	2 - 10	6 - 9
C 16:1 PALMITOLEIC	2 MAX	0 - 8.3			< 0.5	< 1.5		< 1.0				< 0.5		< 1.0	
C 18:0 STEARIC	3 MAX	0.6 - 1.3	0.8 - 2.0	1 - 4	0.5 - 4	1 - 4	1 - 3	1.3 - 6.5	1.2	1 - 3	1 - 10	3.5 - 6	2.0 - 5.5	1 - 10	1 - 3
C 18:1 OLEIC	60 - 78	42 - 81	3 - 6	5 - 8	19 - 50	13 - 44	65 - 85	36 - 72	61	40 - 50	7 - 42	35 - 50	19 - 30	14 - 65	15 - 25
C 18:2 LINOLEIC	10 - 30	6 - 18.5	3.5 - 6.8	2.5 MAX	34 - 65	40 - 63	4 - 15	13 - 45	30	29 - 42	72 - 81	35 - 50	48 - 58	20 - 75	> 50

1 From bibliography reference no. 32.

	ALMOND	AVOCADO	CASTOR	COCONUT	CORN	COTTON-SEED	OLIVE	PEANUT	PERSIC	RICE BRAN	SAF-FLOWER	SEASAME	SOYBEAN	SUN-FLOWER	WALNUT
C 18:3 LINOLENIC	2 MAX	2 MAX			< 2.0	0.1 - 2.1	< 1.5	< 2.0		< 2.0	< 1.5	< 1.0	5 - 9	< 1.5	< 16
C 18:1 RICINOLEIC			82 - 95												
C 20:0 ARACHIDIC				0.4 MAX	< 1.0	0.5 MAX		1 - 2.5		< 2.5	< 0.5	< 1.0	< 1.0	< 1.0	
C 20:1 GADOLEIC					< 0.5	0.5 MAX		0.5 - 2.1			< 0.5	< 0.5	< 1.0	< 0.5	
C 20:4 ARACHIDONIC								1 - 2.5							
C 22:0 BEHENIC						0.5 MAX		1.5 - 4.8				< 0.5		< 1.0	
C 24:0 LIGNOCERIC						< 0.5		1.0 - 2.5	0.1					< 0.5	
COLOR GARDENER (MAX)	4	4	3	3	5	5	8	4	4	4	3	4	4	3	4
ACID VALUE (MAX)	2.8	0.25	2	0.25	0.25	0.25	2.8	0.25	0.25	0.25	0.25	0.25	0.2	0.25	0.2
IODINE VALUE (HANUS)	95 - 105	71 - 95	83 - 88	6 - 11	102 - 130	109 - 120	79 - 88	84 - 100	90 - 108	99 - 108	135 - 150	103 - 116	120 - 143	110 - 143	140 - 162
SAPONIFICATION VALUE	190 - 200	177 - 196	176 - 182	250 - 264	187 - 193	190 - 198	190 - 195	185 - 195	185 - 195	181 - 189	186 - 194	188 - 195	180 - 200	188 - 194	190 - 197
SPECIFIC GRAVITY 25°C	0.910 - 0.915	0.910 - 0.916	0.957 - 0.961	0.917 - 0.922	0.914 - 0.921	0.915 - 0.921	0.910 - 0.915	0.912 - 0.920	0.910 - 0.923	0.916 - 0.921	0.919 - 0.924	0.916 - 0.921	0.917 - 0.921	0.915 - 0.920	0.920 - 0.928

Appendix C
Worldwide Sunscreen Approved Ingredients[1]

Country and Use Percent Approved

INCI Designation	US	Japan	EU
3-Benzylidene Camphor			2
4-Methylbenzlidene Camphor			4
Benzophenone-1		10	
Benzophenone-2		10	
Benzophenone-3	6	5	10
Benzophenone-4	10	10	5
Benzophenone-5		10	
Benzophenone-6		10	
Benzophenone-8	3		
Benzophenone-9		10	
Benzylidine Camphor Sulfonic Acid			6
Butyl Methoxydibenzoylmethane	3	10	5
Camphor Benzalkonium Methosulfate			6
Cinoxate	3	5	
Diethylhexyl Butamido Triazone			10
Diisopropyl Methyl Cinnamate		10	
Dipropylene Glycol Salicylate		0.2	
Drometrizole Trisiloxane			15
Ethyl PABA		4	
Ethylhexyl Dimethyl PABA	8	10	8

---

1   From bibliography reference no. 29.

INCI Designation	US	Japan	EU
Ethylhexyl Methoxycinnamate	7.5	10	10
Ethylhexyl Salicylate	5	10	5
Ethylhexyl Triazone		3	5
Glyceryl Ethylhexanoate Dimethoxycinnamate		10	
Glyceryl PABA		4	
Homosalate	15	10	10
Isoamyl p-Methoxycinnamate			10
Isopropyl Methoxycinnamate		10	
Menthyl Anthranilate	5		
Octocrylene	10		10
PABA	15	4	5
PEG-25 PABA			10
Phenylbenzimidazole Sulfonic Acid	4		8
Polyacrylamidomethyl Benzylidene Camphor			6
TEA-Salicylate	12		
Terephthalylidene Dicamphor Sulfonic Acid			10
Titanium Dioxide	25	no limit	no limit
Zinc Oxide	25	no limit	no limit

Appendix D
Common Denaturants for
"Specially Denatured" Alcohol
(A.K.A. SD Alcohol)

Formula No. 1.
Formula. To every 100 gallons of alcohol add:
Four gallons of methyl alcohol and either 1/8 avoirdupois ounce of denatonium benzoate, N.F., (BITREX); 1 gallon of methyl isobutyl ketone; 1 gallon of mixed isomers of nitropropane; or 1 gallon of methyl *n*-butyl ketone.

Formula No. 2-B.
Formula. To every 100 gallons of alcohol add:
One-half gallon of benzene, ½ gallon of rubber hydrocarbon solvent, or ½ gallon of toluene.

Formula No. 2-C.
Formula. To every 100 gallons of alcohol add:
Thirty-three pounds or more of metallic sodium and either ½ gallon of benzene, ½ gallon of toluene, or ½ gallon of rubber hydrocarbon solvent.

Formula No. 3-A.
Formula. To every 100 gallons of alcohol add:
Five gallons of methyl alcohol.

Formula No. 3-B.
Formula. To every 100 gallons of alcohol add:
One gallon of pine tar, U.S.P.

Formula No. 3-C.
Formula. To every 100 gallons of alcohol add:
Five gallons of isopropyl alcohol.

Formula No. 4.
Formula. To every 100 gallons of alcohol, or to every 100 gallons of rum of not less than 150 proof, add:
One gallon of the following solution: Five gallons of an aqueous solution containing 40 percent nicotine; 3.6 avoirdupois ounces of methylene blue, U.S.P.; and water sufficient to make 100 gallons.

Formula No. 6-B.

Formula. To every 100 gallons of alcohol add:
One-half gallon of pyridine bases.

Formula No. 12-A.

Formula. To every 100 gallons of alcohol add:
Five gallons of benzene, or five gallons of toluene.

Formula No. 13-A.

Formula. To every 100 gallons of alcohol add:
Ten gallons of ethyl ether.

Formula No. 17.

Formula. To every 100 gallons of alcohol add:
Five-hundredths (0.05) gallon (6.4 fluid ounces) of
bone oil (Dipple's oil).

Formula No. 18.

Formula. To every 100 gallons of alcohol of not less than 160
proof, add:
One hundred gallons of vinegar of not less than 90-
grain strength or 150 gallons of vinegar of not less
than 60-grain strength.

Formula No. 19.

Formula. To every 100 gallons of alcohol add:
One hundred gallons of ethyl ether.

Formula No. 20.

Formula. To every 100 gallons of alcohol add:
Five gallons of chloroform.

Formula No. 22.

Formula. To every 100 gallons of alcohol add:
Ten gallons of formaldehyde solution, U.S.P.

Formula No. 23-A.

Formula. To every 100 gallons of alcohol add:
Eight gallons of acetone, U.S.P.

Formula No. 23-F.

Formula. To every 100 gallons of alcohol add:
Three pounds of salicylic acid, U.S.P., 1 pound of resor-
cinol (resorcin), U.S.P., and 1 gallon of bergamot oil,
N.F. XI, or bay oil (myrcia oil), N.F. XI.

Formula No. 23-H

Formula. To every 100 gallons of alcohol add:
Eight gallons of acetone, U.S.P., and 1.5 gallons of methyl isobutyl ketone.

Formula No. 25.

Formula. To every 100 gallons of alcohol add:
Twenty pounds of iodine, U.S.P., and 15 pounds of either potassium iodide, U.S.P., or sodium iodide, U.S.P.

Formula No. 25-A.

Formula. To every 100 gallons of alcohol add:
A solution composed of 20 pounds of iodine, U.S.P.; 15 pounds of either potassium iodide, U.S.P., or sodium iodine, U.S.P.; and 15 pounds of water.

Formula No. 27.

Formula. To every 100 gallons of alcohol add:
One gallon of rosemary oil, N.F. XII, and 30 pounds of camphor, U.S.P.

Formula No. 27-A.

Formula. To every 100 gallons of alcohol add:
Thirty-five pounds of camphor, U.S.P., and 1 gallon of clove oil, N.F.

Formula No. 27-B

Formula. To every 100 gallons of alcohol add:
One gallon of lavender oil, N.F., and 100 pounds of green soap, U.S.P.

Formula No. 28-A.

Formula. To every 100 gallons of alcohol add:
One gallon or any combination totaling one gallon of either gasoline, unleaded gasoline, heptane, or rubber hydrocarbon solvent.

Formula No. 29.

Formula. To every 100 gallons of alcohol add:
One gallon of 100 percent acetaldehyde or 5 gallons of an alcohol solution of acetaldehyde containing not less than 20 percent acetaldehyde, or 1 gallon of ethyl acetate having as ester content of 100 percent, or, where approved by the appropriate ATF officer as to material and quantity, not less than 6.8 pounds if solid, or 1 gallon if liquid, of any chemical. When material other than acetaldehyde or ethyl acetate is proposed to be used, the user shall submit an application for such to the Chief, Chemical Branch. The application shall include specifications, assay methods, and an 8-ounce sample of the substitute material for analysis.

Formula No. 30.
> *Formula.* To every 100 gallons of alcohol add:
> Ten gallons of methyl alcohol.

Formula No. 31-A.
> *Formula.* To every 100 gallons of alcohol add:
> One hundred gallons of glycerin (glycerol), U.S.P., and 20 pounds of hard soap, N.F. XI.

Formula No. 32.
> *Formula.* To every 100 gallons of alcohol add:
> Five gallons of ethyl ether.

Formula No. 33.
> *Formula.* To every 100 gallons of alcohol add:
> Thirty pounds of gentian violet or gentian violet, U.S.P.

Formula No. 35.
> *Formula.* To every 100 gallons of alcohol add:
> 29.75 gallons of ethyl acetate having an ester content of 100 percent by weight or the equivalent thereof not to exceed 35 gallons of ethyl acetate with an ester content of not less than 85 percent by weight.

Formula No. 35-A.
> *Formula.* To every 100 gallons of alcohol add:
> 4.25 gallons of ethyl acetate having an ester content of 100 percent by weight or the equivalent thereof not to exceed 5 gallons of ethyl acetate with an ester content of not less than 85 percent by weight.

Formula No. 36.
> *Formula.* To every 100 gallons of alcohol add:
> Three gallons of ammonia, aqueous, 27 to 30 percent by weight; 3 gallons of strong ammonia solution, N.F.; 17.5 pounds of caustic soda, liquid grade, containing 50 percent sodium hydroxide by weight; or 12.0 pounds of caustic soda, liquid grade, containing 73 percent sodium hydroxide by weight.

Formula No. 37.
> *Formula.* To every 100 gallons of alcohol add:
> Forty-five fluid ounces of eucalyptol, N.F. XII, 30 avoirdupois ounces of thymol, N.F., and 20 avoirdupois ounces of menthol, U.S.P.

Formula No. 38-B.

Formula. To every 100 gallons of alcohol add:
Ten pounds of any one, or a total of 10 pounds of two or more, of the oils and substances listed below:

Alpha Terpineol
Anethole, N.F.
Anise Oil, N.F.
Bay oil (myrcia oil) N.F. XI.
Benzaldehyde, N.F.
Bergamot oil, N.F. XI.
Bitter almond oil, N.F. X.
Camphor, U.S.P.
Cedar leaf oil, U.S.P. XIII.
Chlorothymol, N.F. XII.
Cinnamic aldehyde, N.F. IX.
Cinnamon oil, N.F.
Citronella oil, natural.
Clove oil, N.F.
Coal tar, U.S.P.
Eucalyptol, N.F. XII.
Eucalyptus oil, N.F.
Eugenol, U.S.P.
Guaiacol, N.F. X.
Lavender oil, N.F.
Menthol, U.S.P.

Methyl salicylate, N.F.
Mustard oil, volatile (allyl isothiocyanate), U.S.P. XII.
Peppermint oil, N.F.
Phenol, U.S.P.
Phenyl salicylate (salol), N.F. XI.
Pine oil, N.F. XII.
Pine needle oil, dwarf, N.F.
Rosemary oil, N.F. XII.
Safrole.
Sassafras oil, N.F. XI.
Spearmint oil, N.F.
Spearmint oil, terpeneless.
Spike lavender oil, natural.
Storax, U.S.P.
Thyme oil, N.F. XII.
Thymol, N.F.
Tolu balsam, U.S.P.
Turpentine Oil, N.F. XI.

Formula No. 38-C.

Formula. To every 100 gallons of alcohol add:
Ten pounds of menthol, U.S.P., and 1.25 gallons of formaldehyde solution, U.S.P.

Formula No. 38-D.

Formula. To every 100 gallons of alcohol add:
Two and one-half pounds of menthol, U.S.P., and 2.5 gallons of formaldehyde solution, U.S.P.

Formula No. 38-F

Formula. To every 100 gallons of alcohol add:
1.   Six pounds of either boric acid, N.F., or Polysorbate 80, N.F.; 1-1/3 pounds of thymol, N.F.; 1 1/3 pounds of chlorathymol, N.F. XII; and 1-1/3 pounds of menthol, U.S.P.; or
2.   A total of at least 3 pounds of any two or more denaturing materials listed under Formula No. 38-B,

plus sufficient boric acid, N.F., or Polysorbate 80, N.F., to total 10 pounds of denaturant; or

3.   Seven pounds of zinc chloride, U.S.P., 2.6 fluid ounces of hydrochloric acid, N.F., and a total of 3 pounds of any two or more of the denaturing materials listed under Formula No. 38-B.

Formula No. 39.

Formula. To every 100 gallons of alcohol add:
Nine pounds of sodium salicylate, U.S.P., or salicylic acid, U.S.P.; 1.25 gallons of fluid extract of quassia, N.F. VII; and 1/8 gallon of *tert*-butyl alcohol.

Formula No. 39-A.

Formula. To every 100 gallons of alcohol add:
Sixty avoirdupois ounces of any one of the following alkaloids or salts together with 1/8 gallon of *tert*-butyl alcohol:

Quinine, N.F. X.
Quinine bisulfate, N.F. XI.
Quinine dihydrochloride, N.F. XI.
Cinchonidine.
Cinchonidine sulfate, N.F. IX.

Formula No. 39-B.

Formula. To every 100 gallons of alcohol add:
Two and one-half gallons of diethyl phthalate and 1/8 gallon of *tert*-butyl alcohol.

Formula No. 39-C.

Formula. To every 100 gallons of alcohol add:
One gallon of diethyl phthalate.

Formula No. 39-D

Formula. To every 100 gallons of alcohol add:
One gallon of bay oil (myrcia oil), N.F. XI, and either 50 avoirdupois ounces of quinine sulfate, U.S.P., 50 avoirdupois ounces of sodium salicylate, U.S.P.

Formula No. 40.

Formula. To every 100 gallons of alcohol add 1/8 gallon of *tert-butyl alcohol add:*
One and one-half avoirdupois ounces of either (1) brucine alkaloid, (2) brucine sulfate, N.F. IX, (3) quassin, or (4) any combination of two or of three of those denaturants.

Formula No. 40-A.

Formula. To every 100 gallons of alcohol add:
One pound of sucrose octaacetate and 1/8 gallon of *tert*-butyl alcohol.

Formula No. 40-B.

Formula. To every 100 gallons of alcohol add:
One sixteenth avoirdupois of denatonium benzoate, N.F. (BITREX), and 1/8 gallon of *tert*-butyl alcohol.

Formula No. 40-C.

Formula. To every 100 gallons of alcohol add:
Three gallons of *tert*-butyl alcohol.

Formula No. 42.

Formula. To every 100 gallons of alcohol add:
1. Eighty grams of potassium iodide, U.S.P., and 109 grams of red mercuric iodide, N.F. XI; or
2. Ninety-five grams of thimerosal, U.S.P.; or
3. Seventy-six grams of any of the following: phenyl mercuric nitrate, N.F.; phenyl mercuric chloride, N.F., IX.; or phenyl mercuric benzoate.

Formula No. 45.

Formula. To every 100 gallons of alcohol add:
Three hundred pounds of refined white or orange shellac.

Formula No. 46.

Formula. To every 100 gallons of alcohol add:
Twenty-five fluid ounces of phenol, U.S.P., and 4 fluid ounces of methyl salicylate, N.F.

Bibliography

1. *The Merck Index;* Eleventh Edition, Merck & Co., Inc., Rahway, NJ, U.S.A., 1989.
2. Alexander, P., et al., *Harry's Cosmeticology,* New York, NY, Chemical Publishing, 1982.
3. de NaVarre, M.G., *The Chemistry and Manufacture of Cosmetics—Volume IV,* Orlando, FL, Continental Press, 1975.
4. Grieve, M., *A Modern Herbal,* Chatham, Kent, England, Barnes and Noble, 1996.
5. Bashier, S., Compound Allergy, *Cosmetics and Toiletries Magazine,* Vol. 113, December, 1998.
6. Schueller, R. and Romanowski, P., *Beginning Cosmetic Chemistry,* Carol Stream, IL, Allured Publishing Corp., 1999.
7. *International Journal of Dermatology,* #33, 1994.
8. Hofland, H.E.J., et. al., *Interactions between non-ionic surfactant vesicles and Human Stratum Corneum in-vitro,* J. Liposome Res. 5 241–263, 1995.
9. Tsen-Fang, M.D., *Water: A Possible Skin Irritant,* Cosmetics and Toiletries Magazine, Vol. 115, No. 2, February, 2000.
10. Kim, S. J., et. al., *Skin Pharmacology* 10 (4) 200–205, 1997.
11. Keller, K.L., et. al., *J. Am. Acad. Dermatology* 39:611–625, 1998.
12. Griffith, H.W., M.D., *Vitamins, Herbs, Minerals and Supplements—The Complete Guide,* New York, NY, MJF Books, 1998.
13. Willard, T. Ph.D., *Textbook of Modern Herbology,* Calgary, Alberta, Canada, Progressive Publishing, Inc., 1998.
14. Carr, A., et. al., *Rodale's Illustrated Encyclopedia of Herbs,* Emmus, Penn., Rodale Press, 1987.
15. Stary, F., *Medicinal Herbs and Plants,* New York, NY, Barnes and Noble, 1994.
16. Santillo, H., B.S. MH, *Natural Healing with Herbs,* Prescott, AZ, Hohm Press, 1991.
17. Tyler, V.E., Ph.D., *The Honest Herbal,* Binghamton, NY, 1993.
18. Jellinek, S.J., Dr., *Formulation and Function of Cosmetics,* New York, NY, John Wiley & Sons Inc., 1970.
19. *Federal Register,* Vol. 64, No. 98, Page 27687, May 21, 1999.
20. Corbella, A., *Cosmetic News* 20 (117) 417–421, 1997 (in Italian).

Bibliography

21. Schueller, R. and Romanowski, P., *Understanding Mild Cosmetic Products*, Cosmetics and Toiletries Magazine, Vol. 114, No. 12/ December, 1999.

22. *Feather River Cosmetic Ingredient Glossary*, Feather River Co., Petaluma, CA, 1988.

23. Floyd, D.T., and Howe, A.M., *Alkyl Modified Siloxanes: Key Ingredients for Formula Optimization*, Cosmetics and Toiletries Magazine, pages 51–58, Vol. 115, No. 4, April, 2000.

24. Whalley, G.R., *Chitosan, a Versatile, Natural Ingredient for Personal Care Products*, Happi Magazine, pages 65–68, May, 2000.

25. Giacomoni, P.U., and Maes, D.H., *Sensitive Skin in Different Ethnic Groups*, Multicultural Personal Care, pages 20–23, May, 2000.

26. Fishman, H.M., *Cocoa Butter, How Sweet It Is*, Happi Magazine, page 42, May, 2000.

27. Dowden, B., *Purcell Jojoba International*, (Supplied information on Jojoba products), Avila Beach, CA.

28. McDaniel, D, M.D., *Topical Vitamin C Use—Claims and Controversy*, Cosmetic and Toiletries Magazine, page 100, Vol. 115, No. 4, May, 2000.

29. Steinberg, D., *Encyclopedia of UV Filters Updated*, Cosmetic and Toiletries Magazine, pages 69–75, Vol. 115, No. 4, March, 2000.

30. Tao, L., *Skin Delivery from Lipid Vesicles*, Cosmetic and Toiletries Magazine, pages 43–50, Vol. 115, No. 4, April, 2000.

31. Morganti, P. M.D., *Clinically Correct Cosmetics to Maintain Skin Homeostasis*, www.globalcosmetic.com, pages 32–38, April, 2000.

32. *Fats—Oils—Fatty Acids*, Welch, Holme and Clark Co., Inc., Newark, NJ, 1997.

33. Benzdicek, R., and Lyons, S., *Sodium Lauryl Sulfoacetate for Personal Care Products*, Cosmetics and Toiletries Manufacture Worldwide, pages 123–128, 2000.

34. Djerassi, D., and Hickling, M., *The Role of Vitamins in High Performance Cosmetics*, Cosmetics and Toiletries Manufacture Worldwide, pages 305–311, 2000.

35. D' Amelio, F., Sr., and Mirhom, Y., *Paper Mulberry and its Preparation as Tyrosinase Inhibitors and Skin Lightening Agents*, Cosmetics and Toiletries Manufacture Worldwide, pages 31–34, 2000.

36. Charbonnelle, A., *Enzymes, Skin and Actives for Cosmetology*, Cosmetics and Toiletries Manufacture Worldwide, pages 197–202, 2000.

37. Ash, M., and I., *Handbook of Industrial Surfactants*, Third Edition, Volumes 1 and 2, Synapse Information Resources, Inc., Endicott, NY 13760.

38. Bronaugh, R., and Maibach, H., *Percutaneous Absorption*, Marcel Dekker, New York, NY, 1989.

Bibliography

39. Grove, G.L., Soshin, D.M., and Kligman, A.M., *Adverse Subjective Reactions to Topical Agents*, Cutaneous Toxicology, Raven Press, New York, NY (1984).

40. Draelos, Z. D., *Formulating for Sensitive Skin*, Department of Dermatology, Wake Forest University School of Medicine, Winston-Salem, NC, Cosmetics and Toiletries Magazine, Vol. 115, No. 6, June, 2000.

41. Loiseau, A., and Mercier, M., *Centella Asiatica and Skin Care*, Cosmetics and Toiletries Magazine, pages 63–67, Vol. 115, No. 6, June, 2000.

42. Wincor, M.Z, Pharm. D., BCPP, *Bioflavonoids*, Continuing Education Module, University of Southern California, September, 1999.

43. Silverman, H.M., Pharm. D., Romano, J., Pharm. D., Elmer, G., Ph. D., *The Vitamin Book*, Bantam Books, NY, 1999.

44. Graziano, M., *New Choices in Vegetable-derived Thixotropes for the Oil Phase in Personal Care Applications*, Cosmetics and Toiletries Manufacture Worldwide, pages 57–61, 2000.

45. Gallagher,R., et. al., Cancer Control Research Program, British Columbia Cancer Agency, Journal of the American Medical association, June 14, 2000.

46. Harpin, V., Rutter, N., *Barrier Functions of the Newborn Infant's Skin*, J. Pediatrics, 102, pages 419–425 (1983).

47. Gilchrest, B.A., *Photodamage*, Blackwell Science ed., Oxford, UK, (1995).